OXFORD MEDICAL PUBLICATIONS

Oxfo

Der

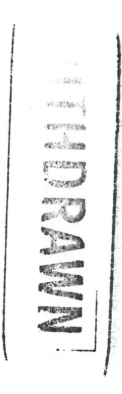

Published and forthcoming Oxford Handbooks in Nursing

Oxford Handbook of Midwifery 2e
Edited by Janet Medforth,
Susan Battersby, Maggie Evans,
Beverley Marsh, and Angela Walker

Oxford Handbook of Adult Nursing
Edited by George Castledine and
Ann Close

Oxford Handbook of Cancer Nursing
Edited by Mike Tadman and
Dave Roberts

Oxford Handbook of Cardiac Nursing
Edited by Kate Johnson and
Karen Rawlings-Anderson

Oxford Handbook of Children's and Young People's Nursing
Edited by Edward Alan Glasper,
Gillian McEwing, and Jim Richardson

Oxford Handbook of Clinical Skills for Children's and Young People's Nursing
Edited by Paula Dawson, Louise
Cook, Laura-Jane Holliday, and
Helen Reddy

Oxford Handbook of Clinical Skills in Adult Nursing
Edited by Jacqueline Randle, Frank
Coffey, and Martyn Bradbury

Oxford Handbook of Critical Care Nursing
Sheila K Adam and Sue Osborne

Oxford Handbook of Dental Nursing
Edited by Elizabeth Boon, Rebecca
Parr, Dayananda Samarawickrama,
and Kevin Seymour

Oxford Handbook of Diabetes Nursing
Edited by Lorraine Avery and
Sue Beckwith

Oxford Handbook of Emergency Nursing
Edited by Robert Crouch, Alan
Charters, Mary Dawood, and Paula
Bennett

Oxford Handbook of Gastrointestinal Nursing
Edited by Christine Norton, Julia
Williams, Claire Taylor, Annmarie
Nunwa, and Kathy Whayman

Oxford Handbook of Learning and Intellectual Disability Nursing
Edited by Bob Gates and Owen Barr

Oxford Handbook of Mental Health Nursing
Edited by Patrick Callaghan and
Helen Waldock

Oxford Handbook of Musculoskeletal Nursing
Edited by Susan Oliver

Oxford Handbook of Neuroscience Nursing
Edited by Sue Woodward and
Catheryne Waterhouse

Oxford Handbook of Nursing Older People
Edited by Beverley Tabernacle, Marie
Honey, and Annette Jinks

Oxford Handbook of Orthopaedic and Trauma Nursing
Rebecca Jester, Julie Santy, and Jean
Rogers

Oxford Handbook of Perioperative Practice
Edited by Suzanne Hughes and Andy
Mardell

Oxford Handbook of Prescribing for Nurses and Allied Health Professionals 2e
Edited by Sue Beckwith and Penny
Franklin

Oxford Handbook of Primary Care and Community Nursing
Edited by Vari Drennan and Claire
Goodman

Oxford Handbook of Respiratory Nursing
Edited by Terry Robinson and Jane
Scullion

Oxford Handbook of Women's Health Nursing
Edited by Sunanda Gupta, Debra
Holloway, and Ali Kubba

Oxford Handbook of
Dental
Nursing

Edited by

Elizabeth Boon

Quality Assurance Auditor
National Examination Board for Dental Nurses Fleetwood

Rebecca Parr

Dental Nurse Training Manager Barts and The London
School of Medicine and Dentistry Queen Mary,
University of London, London

Dayananda Samarawickrama

Honorary Consultant in Restorative Dentistry
Barts and The London School of Medicine and Dentistry
London, UK

Kevin Seymour

Senior Lecturer and Honorary Consultant
Barts and The London School of Medicine and Dentistry
London, UK

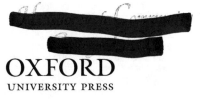

OXFORD
UNIVERSITY PRESS

OXFORD
UNIVERSITY PRESS

Great Clarendon Street, Oxford, OX2 6DP,
United Kingdom

Oxford University Press is a department of the University of Oxford.
It furthers the University's objective of excellence in research, scholarship,
and education by publishing worldwide. Oxford is a registered trade mark of
Oxford University Press in the UK and in certain other countries

© Oxford University Press 2012

Published in the United States of America by Oxford University Press
198 Madison Avenue, New York, NY 10016, United States of America

British Library Cataloguing in Publication Data
Data available

Library of Congress Cataloging in Publication Data
Oxford Handbook of dental nursing / edited by Elizabeth Boon … [et al.].
P. ; cm.—(Oxford handbooks)
Includes bibliographical references and index.
ISBN 978–0–19–923590–2 (alk. Paper)
I. Boon, Elizabeth. II. Series: Oxford Handbooks.
[DNLM: 1. Dental Assistants-Handbooks. 2. Dentistry-methods-Handbooks.
WU 49]
LC classification not assigned
617.6'0233-dc23   2011033030

Preface

Since the introduction of mandatory General Dental Council registration in 2008, the role of the dental nurse and the theoretical and practical training required in order to become a qualified dental nurse have evolved greatly. Registration has brought about extended duties for the dental nurse, which in practice has allowed dental nurses to continue to develop their skills further after registration and contribute more to the care and treatment of patients.

The aim of the *Oxford Handbook of Dental Nursing* is to provide a practical, easily accessible book for student dental nurses who are completing their initial training qualification and as a reference tool for qualified dental nurses, in an easily portable format. Those who are involved in the training and development of dental nurses, especially those new to the role, can use this book to gauge the depth of knowledge required by the dental nurse and the various areas of study which need to be covered. The handbook will enable users to find relevant information quickly and is small enough to be carried in a uniform pocket or in a student's, tutor's, mentor's or supervisor's bag without taking up valuable space.

The book has been written and edited by a combination of dental professionals who have experience working at the chair side, those who have had some experience of training dental nurses, and those who work in specialized areas of dentistry. In addition to the traditional topics addressed in a dental nursing textbook, there are extra chapters which cover the behaviour expected of a registered dental nurse, advice on applying for jobs, writing a curriculum vitae, and what to expect at an interview.

Thanks are expressed to all those who have been involved in the book, but extra thanks should be reserved for Mrs Caroline Zuber who entrusted her team to undertake this task.

Contents

Contributors

Katharine Bond
DCP Training Co-ordinator
King's College Dental Hospital
London

Elizabeth Boon
Quality Assurance Auditor
National Examination Board for
Dental Nurses
Fleetwood

John Buchanan
Clinical Senior Lecturer/
Honorary Consultant and
Clinical Lead for Oral Medicine
Barts and The London School of
Medicine and Dentistry
Queen Mary, University of London
London

David O'Donnell
Associate Specialist in Paediatric
Dentistry, Hon Clinical Senior
Lecturer, Barts and The London
School of Medicine and Dentistry
Queen Mary, University of London
London

Padhraig S. Fleming
Locum Consultant Orthodontist
Barts and The London School of
Medicine and Dentistry
Queen Mary, University of London
London

Ama Johal
Senior Lecturer/Consultant
Orthodontist
Barts and The London School of
Medicine and Dentistry
Queen Mary, University of London
London

Helen Liversidge
Senior Clinical Lecturer
Barts and The London School of
Medicine and Dentistry
Queen Mary, University of London
London

Robert McGeoch
Clinical Senior Lecturer/Honorary
Consultant
Barts and The London School of
Medicine and Dentistry
Queen Mary, University of London
London

Christopher Mercer
Hon Senior Lecturer and
Hon Consultant in Restorative
Dentistry
Centre for Adult Oral Health
Barts and The London School of
Medicine and Dentistry
Queen Mary, University of London
London

Hitesh Mody
Clinical Tutor and General
Dental Practitioner
Barts and The London School
of Medicine and Dentistry
Queen Mary, University of London
London

Rebecca Parr
Dental Nurse Training Manager
Barts and The London School of
Medicine and Dentistry
Queen Mary, University of London
London

Saman Warnakulsuriya
Professor and Honorary
Consultant, Oral Medicine
and Experimental Oral
Pathology
King's College London
London

Symbols and Abbreviations

►	important
❶	warning
📖	cross-reference
↑	increase/d
↓	decrease/d
>	greater than
<	less than
∴	therefore
♂	male
♀	female
1°	primary
2°	secondary
°	degrees
℘	website
AUG	acute ulcerative gingivitis
BPE	basic periodontal examination
BSE	bovine spongiform encephalopathy
CDT	clinical dental technician
CertHE	Certificate of Higher Education
CJD	Creutzfeldt–Jakob disease
COSHH	Control of Substances Hazardous to Health
CPD	continuing professional development
CPR	cardiopulmonary resuscitation
CT	computed tomography
DCP	dental care professional
ECG	electrocardiogram
FDI	International Dental Federation
FNA	fine-needle aspiration
GA	general anaesthesia
GDC	General Dental Council
GP	gutta-percha or general practitioner
GTN	glyceryl trinitrate
ID	inferior dental
IM	intramuscular
INR	international normalized ratio
IS	inhalation sedation

IV	intravenous
LA	local anaesthesia
MRI	magnetic resonance imaging
NEBDN	National Examination Board for Dental Nurses
NHS	National Health Service (UK)
NiTi	nickel–titanium
NVQ	National Vocational Qualification
OSCE	objective structured clinical examination
PPE	personal protective equipment
RCT	root-canal treatment or therapy
RIDDOR	Reporting of Injuries, Diseases, and Dangerous Occurrences Regulations
SLS	sodium lauryl sulphate
SVQ	Scottish Vocational Qualification
TB	tuberculosis
TMJ	temporomandibular joint
VRQ	Vocationally Related Qualification
WHO	World Health Organization
ZNO	zinc oxide and eugenol

Chapter 1

Becoming a dental nurse

The role of the dental nurse

Although the reception staff are normally the patient's first point of contact in the dental practice, the dental nurse is quite often the first person the patient comes into contact with in the clinical area.

According to the General Dental Council's (GDC) document *Scope of Practice*,[1] dental nurses are registered dental professionals who provide clinical and other support to other registrants and patients.

Dental nurses:
- Prepare and maintain the clinical environment, including the equipment.
- Carry out infection-control procedures to prevent physical, chemical, and microbiological contamination in the surgery or laboratory.
- Record dental charting carried out by other appropriate registrants.
- Prepare, mix, and handle dental materials.
- Provide chairside support to the operator during treatment.
- Keep full and accurate patient records.
- Prepare equipment, materials, and patients for dental radiography.
- Process dental radiographs.
- Monitor, support, and reassure patients.
- Give appropriate advice to patients.
- Support the patient and their colleagues if there is a medical emergency.
- Make appropriate referrals to other health professionals.

This list of duties is taken from the GDC's *Scope of Practice* document.[1]

Personal qualities

A dental nurse should posses certain personal qualities, such as:
- Good written and verbal communication skills.
- The ability to stay calm under pressure.
- A pleasant and caring disposition.
- Excellent attendance, time keeping, and punctuality.
- The ability to work as part of a team.

[1] General Dental Council (2009). *Scope of Practice*. London: GDC. Available at: ⌖ http://www.gdc-uk.org/newsandpublications.

The dental team

There are many different members of the dental team who all have different roles. The members of the team you work with will depend on the environment in which you work. A small practice might have just one dentist, a dental nurse, and a receptionist, whereas a large practice might have many dentists and nurses, a practice manager, hygienists, therapists, and, possibly, their own technicians. By contrast, a hospital environment has a large number of staff, including students, those studying for higher qualifications, and specialists. The GDC recognizes the following members of the dental team who all have different roles, outlined in their *Scope of Practice* document.[1] These are:

- Dental nurses.
- Orthodontic therapists.
- Dental hygienists.
- Dental therapists.
- Dental technicians.
- Clinical dental technicians.
- Dentists.

The following duties and definitions of each professional are from the GDC's *Scope of Practice*.[1]

Orthodontic therapists

An orthodontic therapist is a registered dental professional, who is able to carry out certain aspects of orthodontic treatment under the prescription of a dentist.

Dental hygienists

A dental hygienist is a registered dental professional, who is able to help patients maintain oral health through prevention and treatment of gum disease and oral health promotion. This treatment must be carried out under the prescription of a dentist.

Dental therapists

A dental therapist is a registered dental professional, who is able to carry out certain items of treatment under the prescription of a dentist. They are able to perform the duties of a hygienist and, in addition, are able to:

- Carry out direct restorations on permanent and primary teeth.
- Carry out pulpotomies on primary teeth.
- Extract primary teeth.
- Place pre-formed crowns on primary teeth.
- Plan the delivery of a patient's care.

Dental technicians

A dental technician is a registered dental professional, who is able to make dental appliances such as dentures, crowns. and bridges under the prescription of a dentist or clinical dental technician. They are also able to repair dentures directly for members of the public.

Clinical dental technicians

A clinical dental technician (CDT) is a registered dental professional who is able to provide complete dentures direct to patients and other dental appliances under the prescription of a dentist. Their qualification as a CDT usually follows initial qualification as a dental technician. CDTs are only able to treat patients who do not have any natural teeth or implants. Patients who do have natural teeth or implants have to be seen by a dentist for a treatment plan, prior to treatment by a CDT. If a CDT is concerned about a patient's oral health, then they will refer the patient to a dentist.

Dentists

A dentist is a registered dental professional who is able to undertake all of the duties and treatments listed for the other groups of professionals, as well as being able to:

- Diagnose disease.
- Prepare comprehensive treatment plans and be responsible for the treatment provided by dental care professionals (DCPs) on their prescription.
- Prescribe and provide endodontic treatment on adult teeth.
- Prescribe and provide fixed orthodontic treatment.
- Prescribe and provide fixed and removable prostheses.
- Carry out oral surgery.
- Carry out periodontal surgery.
- Extract permanent teeth.
- Prescribe and provide crowns and bridges.
- Carry out treatment on patients who are under general anaesthesia.
- Give inhalational and intravenous conscious sedation.
- Prescribe drugs as part of dental treatment.
- Prescribe and interpret radiographs.

For further details about the roles of the various members of the dental team, refer to the GDC's *Scope of Practice*.[1]

There are also a number of other members of the team who at present are not required to be registered.

Receptionist

Training

A dental receptionist is not currently required to have a specific qualification. Some individuals have previous dental nursing experience, which helps when discussing treatment costs and booking appointments, but it is not essential.

Responsibilities

The receptionist is more often than not the first point of contact for the patient in the dental practice. They are responsible for the following:

- Booking appointments.
- Organizing the appointment book.
- Dealing with patients face to face, over the telephone, or by letter/ email.
- Filing and retrieving notes.
- Sending recalls.
- Receiving and calculating payments.

Depending on the practice, the receptionist might also take and place orders, deal with sales representatives, and organize staff rotas.

Practice manager

Training

The dental practice manager is an individual who ensures that the non-clinical duties of running a dental practice are maintained and managed. Although it is not essential for this individual to have dental experience, it might be advantageous when dealing with particular tasks, such as ordering stock.

Responsibilities

The dental practice manager might be responsible for the general day-to-day management of the practice, including the following:
- Health and safety.
- Employing staff.
- Managing financial arrangements.
- Managing information technology.
- Marketing the dental surgery.

Many dental nurses consider the move from dental nurse to dental practice manager a promotion, although they might maintain some clinical duties. These duties will depend on the individual dental practice and staffing levels. The dental practice manager tends to work with all members of the dental team, at different times.

[1] General Dental Council (2009). *Scope of Practice*. London: GDC. Available at: ℘ http://www.gdc-uk.org/newsandpublications.

Compulsory registration

The past: registering on a voluntary basis

For many years, dental nurses could join the register on a voluntary basis. This meant that dental nurses could work in surgeries regardless of their previous training and experience.

The present: requirements from July 2008

An unqualified dental nurse cannot now join the register on the basis of experience alone. Dental nurses must register with the GDC, which requires an approved qualification.

Compulsory registration has given appropriate professional status to dental nurses. That status is not without responsibilities though, including an awareness and knowledge of legal and ethical considerations. It also places certain responsibilities on the registered DCP regarding their professional and personal conduct and obliges them to keep up to date through continuing professional development (CPD). Because of these responsibilities, all dental professionals should be aware of the GDC document *Standards for Dental Professionals* available from the GDC and their website.[1]

There are various types of recognized qualifications available (Table 1.1), depending on where training is undertaken or the format training takes.

Table 1.1 Recognized dental nursing qualifications

Qualification	Awarding body	Further information
National Certificate in Dental Nursing	National Examination Board for Dental Nurses (NEBDN)	http://www.nebdn.org
National Vocational Qualification (NVQ)/ Vocationally Related Qualification (VRQ) in Oral Health Care (level 3) or Level 3 Diploma in Dental Nursing (Dec 2010)	City & Guilds	http://www.city-and-guilds.co.uk
Scottish Vocational Qualification (SVQ) in Oral Health Care (level 3)	Scottish Qualifications Authority	http://www.sqa.org.uk
Hospital Diploma in Dental Nursing	Barts and The London School of Medicine and Dentistry	http://www.qmul.ac.uk or http://www.bartsandthelondon.nhs.uk
Certificate of Higher Education (CertHE) in Dental Nursing	The University of Portsmouth and Cardiff University Teeside	http://www.ports.ac.uk http://www.cardiff.ac.uk http://www.tees.ac.uk
Foundation Degree in Dental Nursing	Northampton	http://www.northampton.ac.uk

[1] General Dental Council (2005). *Standards for Dental Professionals*. London: GDC. Available at: http://www.gdc-uk.org/newsandpublications.

National Examination Board for Dental Nurses (NEBDN) national examination

NEBDN

NEBDN are the recognized awarding body for the following UK qualifications:
- National Certificate in Dental Nursing.
- Dental Sedation Nursing.
- Certificate in Oral Health Education.
- Certificate in Orthodontic Nursing.
- Certificate in Dental Radiography.
- Certificate in Special Care Dental Nursing

The panel of examiners consists of registered dental nurses and dentists who have been qualified for a minimum of 4 years and are registered with the GDC. They must also demonstrate an active involvement and commitment to the training and qualification of dental nurses. All examiners must undergo a residential induction and training programme before they are asked to examine.

In conjunction with the GDC, the NEBDN also set the recommended standards for training dental nurses in the UK. A syllabus for each qualification the NEBDN offers can be found on their website.[1]

The examination

The current format is for the examination to be held twice each year, on the 3rd Saturdays of May and November. Components of the examination are outlined as follows:

Written paper

The student has 2 hours to complete the following:
- Multiple-choice questions.
- Short-answer questions.
- A diagram.
- A charting exercise.
- Four conventional type (essay) questions.

Spotter

The spotter test consists of a set of 5 cards, which each show 4 instruments. Students have 1 minute to correctly write down the correct names of instruments on each card.

Practical and oral examination

The student is taken into a room in which there are 2 examiners and the relevant materials/instruments needed for the tasks. The practical test has 2 parts, which are followed by the oral examination.

Wet practical

This involves the correct preparation of a dental material such as a filling material or cement. The student is given a choice of 2 cards each of which has a task written on them and must read the instructions aloud before completing the task. The student must also give the examiner additional spoken information about the material being used.

Dry practical
The dry practical involves the selection of dental instruments. Again, the student must select 1 of 2 cards and complete the task, discussing the use of each instrument as it is selected.

Oral examination
When the student has completed the practical test, they are asked to take a seat at a table opposite the examiners. A range of items commonly used in dentistry is laid out on the table and the examiners will question the student using some of these items.

A total of 13 minutes are allowed for the practical and oral examination, with an average of 5 minutes for the practical tests and 8 minutes for the oral.

▶**Tips**
- Complete all parts of the paper.
- Complete all of the paper in pen—do not use pencil.
- Remember to tell the examiner before starting the practical test *'Please assume I have washed my hands and am wearing my personal protective equipment'*.
- If using abbreviations in written tests, make a note of them on your paper—e.g. SS = stainless steel or FG = friction grip.

Results of the national examination are normally announced some 8 weeks after the examination.

The new national examination
The current format of the national examination is being reviewed and a new format examination will be introduced in November 2011.

The new format will consist of a written assessment which will include a series of multiple choice questions, and extended matching questions followed by a practical OSCE (objective structured clinical examination) style examination. The 2 elements will be held separately on different days. The student is expected to complete the written element first and if the student is successful in the written element they will be entered in to the practical OSCE.

More details regarding the new format of the examination is available on the NEBDN website.[1]

Other approved qualifications

Hospital Diploma in Dental Nursing

This is a qualification which is delivered and awarded by Barts and The London School of Medicine and Dentistry.

Training and assessment is carried out over a 12-month period during which the student is employed by the Dental Hospital. The diploma syllabus has been designed to meet the GDC learning outcomes.

The assessment/examination is carried out over the 12-month period to assess the student's competence. Once the student has successfully completed the prescribed assessment/examinations they are awarded the Hospital Diploma in Dental Nursing.

Dental Nursing NVQ

This qualification is aimed at dental nurses who, along with other members of the dental team, work in a variety of settings including general dental practices, the community dental service, dental and general hospitals, and the armed forces. During training the student carries out a range of duties including reception duties and practice management to maintaining materials and equipment, cross-infection control, support for the patient and the dentist during clinical procedures, and oral health education.

The Dental Nursing NVQ has been designed with the support of the NEBDN to ensure it meets the needs of dental nurses.

In its current format students are required to complete a total of 11 mandatory units and a written examination to gain the full qualification.

In December 2010 City & Guilds replaced the current NVQ with a new version named the Level 3 Diploma in Dental Nursing which is now on the Qualifications and Credits Framework. The new award (based on the GDC curriculum) requires students to complete 15 units and a written examination in order to gain the full qualification.

CertHE Dental Nursing

This is a relatively new method of training dental nurses, which allows the student, upon successful completion, to gain registration as a dental nurse as well as an academic award. Because the CertHE follows an academic framework, a student may choose to further their studies in dental hygiene and therapy.

The course runs for 15 months and is full-time. During the course, the student is required to complete a balanced programme of theoretical and clinical studies, including:
- Academic skills.
- Health, safety, and infection control procedures.
- General and oral anatomy and physiology.
- Human and oral diseases—pathology and microbiology.
- Preparing and maintaining instruments, materials, and equipment necessary for dental procedures.

- Methods of assisting the operator (i.e. dentist or dental therapist) during all patient treatment requirements (e.g. fillings, crowns, bridges, extractions, surgical procedures, and orthodontics).
- Patient-management techniques.
- Preventive dentistry.
- Dental public health.
- Law and ethics.
- Reflective practice and professionalism.
- Processing, mounting, and quality-assurance techniques associated with taking dental radiographs.

General Dental Council (GDC) registration

Having obtained a recognized dental nursing qualification (see Table 1.1), in order to work in the UK as a dental nurse, an individual must be registered with the GDC.

Registration is relatively straightforward, involving the completion of an application form (including proof of qualification, a character reference, and a health declaration) and payment of a registration fee. Registration must be renewed every year. In order to maintain registration, a dental nurse must then:

- Complete 150 hours of CPD over a 5-year period (cycle), of which 50 hours must be verifiable (see 📖 Continuing professional development, p.386).
- Keep a full record of CPD—at the end of each year, the GDC will ask you to complete a declaration of CPD hours and may request your records as evidence. Completion of this annual statement is a legal obligation.

General Dental Council requirements

The GDC requires registered dental professionals to have indemnity, to ensure that a patient can recover any compensation they may be entitled to. This should cover past periods of practice.

The following indemnity arrangements are recognized by the GDC:
- Professional indemnity insurance held by a registered dental professional or their employer.
- NHS indemnity.
- Membership of a dental defence organization.

❶ If you are employed and all the work you do is within this employment, you may be covered by your employer's arrangements. It is your responsibility to check that these arrangements fully cover you for any risks. Check that these arrangements are detailed in your contract of employment.

For more information, please refer to: ♂ http://www.gdc-uk.org.

Legal and ethical issues

General Dental Council (GDC)

The GDC is the organization which regulates dental professionals in the UK.

Structure

Since a major reorganization in 2009, the Council consists of 24 members:
- 12 members of the public, appointed by the Appointments Commission.
- 12 dental professionals appointed by the Commission to include 8 dentists and 4 DCPs.

Aims of the GDC

The GDC[1] works to protect patients and promote confidence in dental professionals by:
- Registering qualified professionals.
- Setting high standards of dental practice and behaviour.
- Quality-assuring dental education.
- Making sure dental professionals keep up to date.
- Helping if you want to make a complaint about a dental professional.

In addition the GDC aims to:
- Work inclusively with others.
- Be accountable.
- Be open and accessible.
- Be professional and business-like.
- Strive to ensure the promotion of equality of opportunity and diversity.

[1] http://www.gdc-uk.org/aboutus

GDC powers under the Dentists Act

The Dentists Act governs the GDC's functions. The current Act was written in 1984 but was modified in 2005, and it is as a result of this modification that the regulation of DCPs has been brought onto a comparable footing with that of dentists. Thus DCPs (like dentists) are required to maintain high standards of professional conduct, with responsibilities to their patients as first priority.

GDC action under the Dentists Act

The GDC take fitness to practise very seriously and can take a number of actions if a registrant's fitness to practise is found to be impaired, or if they are guilty of a criminal offence. The dentist or DCP can be reprimanded, have conditions placed upon their registration, be suspended, or ultimately they can be erased (struck off) from the register.

Impaired fitness to practise

The following are examples where fitness to practise may be considered impaired:

- *Drink and drugs:* Such that professional performance and consequently patient care is compromised (not forgetting that the use of certain substances is illegal and carries the risk of prosecution, a criminal record, and subsequent GDC action!).
- *False certification:* in the past this has involved, for instance, asking someone else to sit examinations for you (this is now more difficult as photographic proof of identity is normally needed before being allowed in to sit an examination).
- *Resuscitation:* it is a requirement that all dental professionals undergo regular resuscitation training. Failure to do so is considered an impairment to practise.
- *Inadequate infection control:* such as not changing gloves in between patients or not sterilizing instruments.
- *Assault:* verbal, physical, or sexual.

In addition, no dental professional should carry out duties, or be asked to carry out duties that are beyond their competence and training.

Further information on these issues can be found on the GDC website (🖰 http://www.gdc-uk.org).

Record keeping: legal requirements

The purpose of a dental record is to provide an up-to-date record/case history of each patient. Such records may vary from practice to practice, however the basic material should be the same. This will include personal details such as name, address, date of birth, and telephone contact number(s). Clinical information will include such things as a diary of treatment, medical history, consent forms, correspondence, accounts, relevant charts, and radiographs along with any other reports.

Although there is no legal requirement under the NHS for dentists to keep records for >2 years after completion of treatment, it is considered best practice for them to be kept for a minimum of 11 years for adults. This recommendation would also be true for private practice.

The Data Protection Act

This obliges the dentist to register under the Act if they keep patient records on either computer or hard copy. The purpose of the Act is to protect patient information, striking a balance between the rights of the individual and the interest of those who may have a legitimate or legal reason to use such personal information. Patient record information must be:
- Accurate.
- Relevant.
- Kept secure.
- Not disclosed to any unauthorised person.

The patient also has a right to access their records. The key to the Act is to keep information **secure** and **confidential**. Any unauthorized disclosure could result in criminal prosecution or compensation payable to the claimant.

Freedom of Information Act

With the implementation of the Freedom of Information Act the patient has a right of access to their records and to correct inaccuracies.

The Freedom of Information Act allows any person to access information such as emails, minutes of meetings, research, or reports held by public authorities. This includes:
- Central and local government.
- Local authorities.
- Hospitals, doctors' surgeries, dentists, pharmacists, and opticians.
- State schools, colleges, and universities.
- Police force and armed services.

In terms of dentists, this Act applies to NHS practitioners only.

The Caldicott Report (December 1997)

This was a review commissioned to make recommendations to improve the way the NHS handled and protected patient information.[1] The Caldicott report identified 6 principles, similar in many respects to the principles outlined in the Data Protection Act. These were:
- Justify the purpose(s) for using patient data.
- Don't use patient-identifiable information unless it is absolutely necessary.

- Use the minimum necessary patient-identifiable information.
- Access to patient-identifiable information should be on a strict need-to-know basis.
- Everyone with access to patient identifiable information should be aware of their responsibilities to maintain confidentiality.
- Understand and comply with the law, in particular the Data Protection Act.

The report is available on the Department of Health website.[1]

▶ Identifying people using dental records

Dental records frequently play an important role as a means of identifying victims of fatal accidents or serious crime (where often teeth are the only things to survive, particularly in cases of fire). A dental chart of the victim can be released on a national database for all dental surgeries to check, and it is not unusual for these to be published in the dental press. All readers of detective fiction will be familiar with such procedures.

---

[1] http://www.dh.gov.uk/en/Publicationsandstatistics/Publications/PublicationsPolicyAndGuidance/DH_4068403

Confidentiality

It must be clearly understood that disclosure of any information to any unauthorized person is forbidden.

Breach of confidentiality constitutes grounds for instant dismissal and subsequent fitness to practise proceedings.

What information is confidential?

Confidential information constitutes anything disclosed to the dentist from the patient, which has a nature of confidence. Such information may relate to a patient's medical or social history. For example, a patient may report that she is pregnant when her medical history is updated. This information is confidential and if disclosed to anyone else is a breach of this confidentiality, even if apparently well intentioned, such as congratulating the patient's partner.

Release of confidential material

Unless there is good reason for the breach in confidentiality the duty never ceases. However, there are certain situations where information can be given:

• If the patient gives explicit consent to disclose information.
• If the patient gives implied consent to give information to relatives.
• If the breach is in the patient's interest (e.g. with young children, where there is risk of harm or self-harm, neglect, abuse, teenage pregnancy).
• If the breach is in society's interest (for dangerous drivers, possible harm to an individual, notifiable diseases). The Court will determine this.
• When the healthcare professional has dual responsibility (e.g. working in the prison service or members of the armed forces, where the duty to the institution comes before the duty to the patient).
• When a Court of Law compels the disclosure of information. This may happen as a result of the:
  • Prevention of Terrorism Act 1974.
  • Police and Criminal Evidence Act 1984.
• To assist in the identification of a driver involved in a road traffic accident under the Road Traffic Act 1988.

► General rules

- Patients should not be discussed among staff, especially in an open area such as the waiting room.
- All conversations with patients should be conducted in private as much as possible.
- Schools and employers have no legal right to know about patients' appointments, unless the patient themselves has consented to this information being passed on.
- All communication should be sent in a sealed envelope addressed specifically to the patient concerned.
- Patients should be informed of what is being released when they have given consent for disclosure.
- Information should be kept confidential even after a patient dies.

Further advice is available in the GDC booklet *Principles of Patient Confidentiality*.[1]

---

[1] General Dental Council (2009). *Principles of Patient Confidentiality*. London: GDC. Available at: ℘ http://www.gdc-uk.org/newsandpublications

Consent

Other than for the most routine dental procedures (such as an examination) for which implied consent is deemed adequate, valid consent must be obtained from the patient. For consent to be valid it must be informed and freely given. The need to gain consent arises from both a moral right and an ethical principle to respect a person's autonomy and right to self-determination.

Types of consent

Implied consent

In very limited circumstances consent may be implied. This may be when a patient seated in the dental chair indicates agreement to an examination by lying in the dental chair and opening their mouth. Consent for other procedures cannot normally be implied. Opening the mouth does not necessarily mean that the patient has understood what the dentist has explained or implied.

Informed consent

The patient must also be aware of the advantages and disadvantages of the proposed treatment so that they can arrive at an informed decision. Patients must be made aware of, and understand, any risks involved. Patients' expectations must also be addressed so that they are fully aware of what the end results will be under the circumstances. Also the cost of any treatment must be discussed as soon as possible with the patient and again agreed upon.

Specific consent

Means that the patient consents expressly to each of the procedures to be undertaken.

Valid consent

For consent to be valid it must be specific, informed, and normally be given by the patient or a parent or guardian (if the patient is aged under 16 years).

The Family Reform Act 1969 provides that any person aged 16 years or over and who is of sound mind may legally give consent to any surgical, medical, or dental treatment.

> **❶ Important points on consent**
>
> Any form of dental treatment or physical contact with the patient undertaken without consent may amount to assault and a breach of the patient's human rights.
>
> A court may award damages for assault, and the GDC may deem this as a breach of their standards.
>
> Consent for dental treatment must be obtained by the clinician treating that patient, under **no** circumstances should a dental nurse do this.

Further advice is available in the GDC booklet *Principles of Patient Consent*.[1]

[1] General Dental Council (2009). *Principles of Patient Consent*. London: GDC. Available at: http://www.gdc-uk.org/newsandpublications

Complaints

Complaints policy for a practice

Patients have the right to complain about any aspect of their care. The GDC requires all practices to have an in-house policy for handling complaints. It is suggested that a specific person is designated within the practice to deal with complaints and that information about the practice's complaints policy is given to patients. In addition, all written complaints should be acknowledged within 10 days and all information should be held in confidence.

Dealing with a verbal complaint

- Conduct discussions in a private area/room away from other patients and staff.
- Use good positive body language and facial expression.
- Allow the patient to describe their complaint without interruption.
- Take notes and summarize and confirm the issues to be addressed.
- Apologize where appropriate.
- Discuss what action is intended and inform the patient when this is carried out.

Dealing with a written complaint

- Acknowledge the complaint within 2 days.
- Investigate the complaint.
- Send a written response within 10 working days.
- Do not apportion blame and make no personal comments.
- Be open but not defensive.
- Offer an apology if appropriate.

Very often patients are happy to accept an apology at this stage and if necessary, this may often avoid complicated and stressful legal involvement.

▶ **Tip**

Good communication skills and an honest, open approach will always help when dealing with what are potentially very stressful situations.

Anatomical structures and systems relevant to dental care

Blood

Blood is a fluid made up of erythrocytes (red blood cells), leucocytes (white blood cells), and thrombocytes transported around the body in a fluid (which is mainly water) called plasma. A newborn baby has ~300mL of blood, whereas an adult has ~4–5L of blood.

Blood is slightly alkaline and should remain at a constant temperature of 37°C.

Blood travels through a network of vessels in the circulatory system, which includes the heart, arteries, arterioles, capillaries, venules, and veins back to the heart and lungs.

Erythrocytes

Erythrocytes are formed in the bone marrow and remain in the blood system for ~120 days. After this time, they are normally trapped in the spleen, where they are broken down. Erythrocytes contain a pigment called 'haemoglobin', which gives blood its red colour. The 1° function of erythrocytes is related to the transportation of oxygen around the body combined with the removal of carbon dioxide through the lungs.

Leucocytes

Leucocytes are subdivided into five different types, the functions of which vary. 1° functions of leucocytes include dealing with infection and removing injured or dead tissue cells. An increase in the amount of leucocytes may indicate that a disease or infection is present.

Thrombocytes

Platelets have an important role in blood coagulation (clotting).

Plasma

The 1° function of plasma is the transportation of these cells. Additional functions include the following:
- Carrying waste products to the kidneys.
- Removing carbon dioxide from the body by carrying the gas to the lungs before it is expelled.
- Carrying hormones to specific areas.
- Containing antibodies which give resistance to disease.
- Participating in the blood clotting process in association with platelets.
- Maintaining body temperature.

The heart

The heart is a relatively small muscular organ situated just behind and slightly left of the breastbone (Fig. 3.1). The primary function of the heart is to pump blood around the body through a network of vessels. Vessels carrying blood away from the heart are called 'arteries' and those that return blood to the heart are called 'veins'. To do this, the heart beats around 70 times per minute (the 'pulse').

The right atrium of the heart receives blood returning from upper and lower parts of the body through the superior and inferior vena cavae, respectively. These vessels collect blood from around the body, which has become deoxygenated (had its oxygen used up, providing 'energy' for the various cells and tissues of the body).The superior vena cava collects deoxygenated blood from the neck, head, and upper limbs, whereas the inferior vena cava brings deoxygenated blood back from the lower part of the body.

Blood is pumped from the right atrium through the tricuspid valve into the right ventricle. Here, the fluid passes into the pulmonary artery, which divides into 2 branches, 1 to each lung.

Blood sent to the lungs is circulated through arterioles (smaller arterial branches) into a vast network of capillaries, where the blood loses carbon dioxide and collects oxygen. Oxygenated blood leaves the capillaries through venules (small veins), which join up into 4 main pulmonary veins, and flows back to the heart.

Oxygenated blood is carried by pulmonary veins to the left atrium, where it is pumped through the mitral valve and into the left ventricle.

Blood leaves the left ventricle through the aortic valve and aorta, which is the largest artery in the body, and begins its journey around the body.

The aorta divides into smaller arteries to supply the body with blood. Arteries further divide into arterioles and then capillaries at their destination, through which oxygen is expelled and carbon dioxide collected. These capillaries join together to form venules (smaller veins) and, after oxygen is deposited, blood travels through these venules to veins that take the blood back to the superior and inferior vena cavae.

Layers of the heart

Endocardium

The endocardium is the innermost lining of the heart and provides a friction-free surface within the chambers of the heart.

Myocardium

The myocardium is the middle, and thickest, layer of the heart and is primarily made up of cardiac muscle, which is a type of muscle only found in the heart.

Pericardium

The pericardium is the outermost layer of the heart and, in turn, consists of 2 layers that cover the heart. The inner layer is made up of cells, which again provide a smooth friction-free surface, whereas the outer layer is a more fibrous structure, which helps to keep the heart in the right position within the chest.

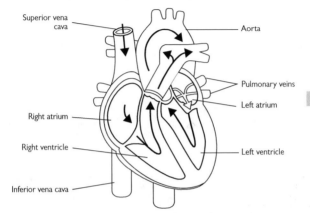

Fig. 3.1 The heart. Reproduced with permission from Johnson K and Rawlings-Anderson K (2007). *Oxford Handbook of Cardiac Nursing*. Oxford: OUP.

The circulatory system

Systemic circulation

The systemic circulation supplies blood to most of the body, apart from those areas discussed in the rest of this topic. Oxygenated blood from the left atrium is pumped through the bicuspid (mitral) valve into the left ventricle. From here, oxygenated blood leaves the heart through the aortic valve and aorta, from which it is distributed around the body by various networks of vessels.

Deoxygenated blood from the head, neck, and upper body returns to the heart through the superior vena cava. Deoxygenated blood from the rest of the body enters the heart through the inferior vena cava. The blood enters the right atrium and is pumped through the tricuspid valve into the right ventricle.

Coronary circulation

As the aorta branches away from the heart, the first branches supply the coronary arteries, which, in turn, supply the walls of the heart. Coronary veins return blood to the right atrium.

Portal circulation

The portal circulation is the blood supply related to the liver. Blood from the stomach, small intestine, colon, and spleen travels through the portal vein within the liver. Deoxygenated blood leaves the liver through the hepatic portal vein, which joins the main circulation.

Pulmonary circulation

Deoxygenated blood is pumped though the right ventricle into the pulmonary artery (see Fig. 3.1) from which it travels to the lungs, where gaseous exchange (loss of carbon dioxide and uptake of oxygen) takes place. Oxygenated blood returns to the heart through the pulmonary vein and into the left atrium. This is the only time that a vein carries oxygenated blood.

Respiration

During respiration, oxygen is taken into the lungs and carbon dioxide is removed. The lungs are situated in the chest, behind the ribcage, and made up of lobes. The right lung has 3 lobes, whereas the left lung only has 2 lobes. This is because the heart is situated just behind and slightly left of the breastbone; the left lung ∴ only has 2 lobes to accommodate the heart.

When a breath is taken, air enters the lungs in 2 ways: through the nose and through the mouth. Air entering the body through the nose undergoes 3 processes (the air is warmed, filtered, and moistened) before joining air that is inhaled through the mouth. The air then travels down the pharynx, into the larynx, and finally into the trachea, which is also known as 'the windpipe'. The air continues its journey into the bronchus and the left and right bronchi. The bronchi subdivide into bronchioles, which, in turn, subdivide into alveoli. Once in the alveoli, the air enters alveolar sacs (Fig. 3.2). These tiny sacs are surrounded by capillaries, where oxygen and carbon dioxide are exchanged.

Mechanism of respiration

The constant expansion and contraction of the lungs ensures that gaseous exchange continues to take place.

External respiration

This is the transport of oxygen from the atmosphere through the lungs into the capillaries, where it is exchanged for carbon dioxide in the blood. Carbon dioxide is then sent from the capillaries through the lungs to the atmosphere.

Internal respiration

This is the transport of oxygen by the blood, from capillaries in the lungs to the various parts of the body. Blood delivers oxygen and picks up carbon dioxide, which it returns to the capillaries.

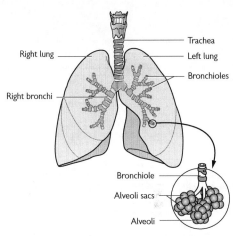

Fig. 3.2 The lungs.

Digestion

Digestion is complex, but the following is a simplistic overview of the process (see Fig. 3.3 for a diagram of the gastrointestinal tract).

Digestion begins with food entering the oral cavity. The food is chewed (or 'masticated'), with the aid of the molar teeth. At the same time, saliva is secreted from the 3 main pairs of salivary glands. Saliva contains an enzyme called 'amylase', which begins digestion of carbohydrates. The food mixed with saliva in addition to the actions of the tongue and muscles of mastication turn the food into a ball known as 'a bolus'.

The tongue pushes the ball to the back of the mouth, where it is swallowed. To prevent food or drink entering the lungs, a small flap known as the epiglottis closes. Food ∴ enters the oesophagus and travels downwards through the contraction and relaxation of the muscles in the oesophagus. Food then enters the stomach through the cardiac sphincter.

In the stomach, another complex process starts, in which food is broken down and mixed with gastric juices and digestive enzymes (pepsin). Food can stay in the stomach for up to 4 hours, after which time it is passed out of the stomach through the pyloric sphincter. Food is further digested in the small intestine.

Finger-like projections called 'villi' are found in the small intestine. Villi are similar to sponges and can soak up large amounts of nutrients from the digested food. From the villi, nutrients flow into the bloodstream and begin their journey through the body.

Waste products that remain after this process are pushed into the large intestine. The waste products ('faeces') remain in the colon for 1–2 days until they are expelled via the anus.

Waste and excess water from the liver are sent to the kidneys. These organs filter out the waste and excess water to produce urine, which is stored in the bladder until it is ready to leave the body.

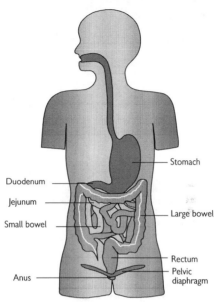

Fig. 3.3 The gastrointestinal system. Reproduced with kind permission © Burdett Institute.

The oral cavity

Similar to the skull, the oral cavity can be difficult to navigate around, especially if using labels on a diagram. Nonetheless, there are certain areas that a dental nurse must be aware of, which are outlined here.

Mucous membrane

The red/pink tissue covering the cheeks, the floor of the mouth and tongue, and the palate is known as 'the mucous membrane'.

Buccal sulcus

The fold between the cheeks and the jaw bones is known as 'the buccal sulcus'.

Palate

The palate is divided into 2 sections:
- The hard palate—a bony area that does not move and is covered by sensitive, but tough, oral mucosa. Small folds of skin known as 'rugae' are found just behind the upper incisors.
- The soft palate—a moveable area that seals off the oral cavity from the nasal cavity during swallowing, to prevent food passing up into the nose.

❶ The gag reflex is a protective mechanism of the soft palate, which keeps foreign objects from entering the trachea. This reflex causes retching and, in some cases, vomiting, so care should be taken during dental treatment to prevent triggering the mechanism. It commonly occurs if the dental nurse is aspirating and touches this sensitive area by mistake.

A cleft palate can occur if the 2 halves of the palate fail to fuse together during development of the fetus.

Tongue

The tongue is a large muscular organ that lies within the mandible. See 📖 The tongue, p.37 for discussion and also Fig. 3.4).

The lingual fraenum is a band of tissue that passes from the underside of the tongue to the floor of the mouth. Similar fraenae are found on the inside of both the lower lip and upper lip.

The tongue

The tongue is a large muscular organ in the floor of the mouth (Fig. 3.4). The top, or dorsal, surface of the tongue is covered by many small projections known as 'papillae'.

Filiform papillae

These are the smallest of the three different types of papillae and found all over the tongue.

Fungiform papillae

These can be found on the top surface and sides of the tongue.

Circumvallate papillae

These are the largest of the different types of papillae and arranged in a 'V-shaped' pattern at the back of the top surface of the tongue.

❶ The tongue is a powerful organ and can sometimes cause problems during aspiration. Care should be taken by the dental nurse not to catch the tongue, but sometimes it cannot be helped.

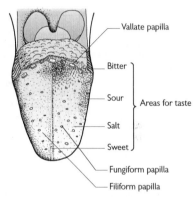

Fig. 3.4 The upper surface of the tongue. Reproduced with permission from Martin EA (ed) (2010). *Concise Oxford Medical Dictionary*. Oxford: OUP.

Saliva and salivary glands

Saliva

Oral tissues are kept moist by saliva, which is a watery secretion from 3 pairs of salivary glands. Saliva is 99.5% water and 0.5% dissolved substances. The human body produces ~1.5L of saliva per day and 45L of saliva per month.

The functions of saliva are as follows:

• Lubricating—saliva lubricates food so that it can be swallowed easily.
• Cleansing—the watery nature of saliva helps clean the mouth by dislodging food debris from around the teeth before being swallowed.
• Digestion—saliva contains an enzyme called 'amylase', which begins digestion of carbohydrates. The water in the saliva enhances the sense of taste.
• Antacid—saliva also helps neutralize acid that causes tooth decay ('caries'). This antacid function of saliva is known as 'a buffer action' and helps the mouth maintain a pH value of 7 (neutral).
• Antibacterial—the mouth is full of germs, most of which are normal and quite harmful. This antibacterial function helps to maintain a good balance of harmless germs and prevent the growth of harmful bacteria.

Salivary glands

Saliva enters the oral cavity through a network of salivary ducts, which, in turn, are connected to a salivary gland. There are 3 main pairs of salivary glands: the parotid, submandibular, and sublingual glands.

Parotid gland

The parotid glands are the largest of the salivary glands. They are situated over the outside, and partly behind, the ramus of the mandible. The parotid duct transports saliva into the oral cavity. The duct passes forwards and then inwards within the cheek, before opening into the buccal sulcus opposite the upper 2nd molar.

The parotid gland is susceptible to viral infections, such as mumps, which causes acute inflammation of the parotid gland.

Submandibular gland

The submandibular glands are found in the floor of the mouth against the inner and lower surface of the angle of the mandible. The submandibular duct passes forwards and into the oral cavity beside the lingual fraenum.

Sublingual gland

The sublingual glands, similar to the submandibular glands, are situated in the floor of the mouth, although much further forwards. Unlike the parotid and submandibular glands, the sublingual glands have many ducts, which open into the floor of the mouth.

The human skull

For any dental nurse, the human skull is a complex area.

The skull can be separated into 4 areas: the mandible, the maxilla, cranial bones, and facial bones (which, to some extent, also form part of the maxilla) (Fig. 3.5).

The $1°$ function of the skull is to protect the brain so, to achieve this, the brain must be protected by a strong outer covering. At birth, the skull has many more bones than it has in later years. Many bones are not fused together so a newborn baby might have ~45 bones. Nevertheless, over time the bones start fusing and are joined together at 'sutures' (a technical anatomical term not to be confused with 'stitches'). When this process has finished, there are ~22 bones.

Cranial bones

In total, there are 8 cranial bones (Table 3.1). These consist of 1 frontal bone, which can be found at the top of the face and forms part of the top of the head.

The 2 parietal bones, 1 on each side, can be found on the side and again on the top of the head. The frontal bone and parietal bones are joined by the coronal suture.

The occipital bone, of which there is 1, can be found at the base of the skull and forms the back of the skull. This is joined to the parietal and temporal bones by the lambdoid suture. The suture joining both parietal bones is known as 'the sagittal suture'.

The 2 temporal bones, again 1 on each side, are located below the parietal bones and form the sides of the head. The sphenoid bone can be found in front of the temporal bone and consists of a body and wings. Lastly, the ethmoid bone lies in the centre of the face and forms part of the nose.

Facial bones

There are 14 facial bones (Table 3.2). The 2 zygomatic bones (or cheek-bones) form part of the cheek. The 2 palatine bones, in turn, form the hard palate of the oral cavity when fused together.

The maxilla is originally made up of 2 bones that fuse together to form 1: the upper jaw. The mandible, or lower jaw, is 1 single bone. The remaining 5 bones are associated with the nose, whereas 2 lacrimal bones can be found behind and to the side of the nasal bones.

Table 3.1 Cranial bones

Name	Position
1 × frontal bone	Top of the face; top part of head
2 × parietal bones	Side and top of the head
2 × temporal bones	Sides of the skull, below the parietal bones, and above and behind the ears
1 × sphenoid bone	In front of the temporal bones; consists of a body and 2 'wings'
1 × occipital bone	Back and base of the cranium; forms the back of the skull
1 × ethmoid bone	Centre of the face, behind the nose

Table 3.2 Facial bones

Name	Position
2 × zygomatic bones	Commonly known as 'the cheekbone' because it forms the prominent part of the cheeks
2 × palatine bones	Bones at the back of the roof of the mouth
2 × nasal bones	2 small bones that form the bridge of the nose and the roof of the nose
1 × maxilla	Forms the upper jaw; 2 halves fuse together
1 × mandible	Known as 'the lower jaw'; the strongest facial bone and the only facial bone that moves
2 × lacrimal bones	Smallest bones in the face; behind and to the side of the nasal bone
2 × inferior nasal conchae	Three thin bones that form the sides of the nasal cavity
1 × vomer	Thin, roughly triangular section of bone on the floor of the nasal cavity that is also part of the nasal septum

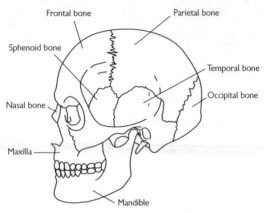

Fig. 3.5 The skull.

The temporomandibular joint

The temporomandibular joint (TMJ) connects the mandible to the rest of the skull near the temporal bone at the side of the head (Fig. 3.6). The mandible should be able to move freely up and down and from side to side with the aid of the muscles of mastication. At rest, the condyle, which is part of the mandible, sits in a hollow within the temporal bone called the 'glenoid fossa'. To stop the bones rubbing together, there is a small disc of fibrous tissue between the glenoid fossa and the condyle.

There is a small ridge in front of the glenoid fossa known as 'the articular eminence', which has an important role when the mandible starts to move.

Mouth opening

When the mouth begins to open, the condyle initially remains in the glenoid fossa. As the mouth opens further, the condyle starts to move downwards and forwards out of the glenoid fossa and onto the articular eminence. When the mouth is fully open, the condyle reaches the crest of the articluar eminence. At this point, the mouth cannot open any further.

The exception is when the mandible becomes dislocated and the condyle slips in front of the articular eminence. This is very painful and might require a general anaesthetic to be reversed.

Mouth closing

When the mouth closes, the whole function is reversed and the condyle returns to its resting position.

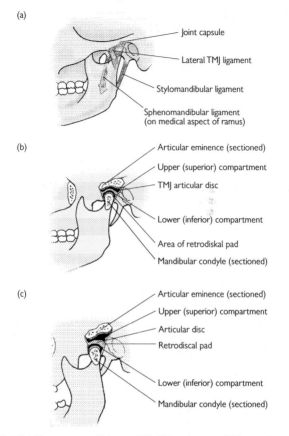

(a)
- Joint capsule
- Lateral TMJ ligament
- Stylomandibular ligament
- Sphenomandibular ligament (on medical aspect of ramus)

(b)
- Articular eminence (sectioned)
- Upper (superior) compartment
- TMJ articular disc
- Lower (inferior) compartment
- Area of retrodiskal pad
- Mandibular condyle (sectioned)

(c)
- Articular eminence (sectioned)
- Upper (superior) compartment
- Articular disc
- Retrodiscal pad
- Lower (inferior) compartment
- Mandibular condyle (sectioned)

Fig. 3.6 a) The temporomandibular joint (TMJ). b) Sagittal section of TMJ—mandible elevated. c) Sagittal section of TMJ—mandible depressed. Reproduced with permission from Scully C (ed) (2003). *Oxford Handbook of Applied Dental Sciences*. Oxford: OUP.

Mastication

Mastication is the chewing of food after it is taken into the mouth. The mouth opens and closes during chewing, with the food held between the upper and lower teeth. The masseter, temporalis, and pterygoid muscles that open and close the mouth by lowering and raising the mandible are called 'muscles of mastication' (Table 3.3).

When food is chewed, it can be shed into the buccal sulcus. The buccinator muscle helps to hold the food between the chewing surfaces of the teeth, so it is considered an accessory muscle of mastication. The buccinator is also considered a muscle of facial expression.

Masseter

The masseter arises from the lower border of the zygomatic arch and is inserted into the outer, or lateral, surface of the ramus of the mandible. It is a very strong and prominent muscle, which is visible on the side of the face, especially when the teeth are clenched.

The muscle raises the mandible. In addition, some parts of the muscle pull the angle of the mandible forwards.

Pterygoids

There are 2 distinct pterygoid muscles: the medial and lateral pterygoid muscles.

Medial pterygoid

The medial pterygoid muscle has 2 origins: 1 from the deep (medial) surface of the pterygoid plate and the other from the maxillary tuberosity and the palatine bone at the base of the skull. The muscle is inserted into the inner (medial) surface of the angle of the mandible.

The muscle pulls the angle of the mandible upwards, forwards, and medially, thus moving the lower jaw towards the opposite side.

Lateral pterygoid

The lateral pterygoid muscle also has 2 origins: 1 from the roof of the infratemporal fossa and the other from the lateral surface of the lateral pterygoid plate (similar to the medial pterygoid muscle). The muscle is inserted into the front of the neck of the mandibular condyle and also the capsule and the interarticular disc of the TMJ.

The muscle pulls the ramus of the mandible and the interarticular disc forwards, thus lowering the jaw and opening the mouth.

Temporalis

The temporalis muscle is 'fan-shaped' and arises from the temporal area of the lateral surface of the skull, above and in front of the ear. The muscle fibres converge and are inserted into the deep (medial) surface of the coronoid process of the mandible.

The muscle raises the mandible and closes the mouth. The muscle also pulls the mandible backwards, in an opposite fashion, to the pterygoid muscles.

Buccinator

The buccinator muscle is 'sheet-like', with 2 opposing sides of the sheet attached to both the maxilla and the mandible, opposite the molar teeth. The posterior border of the muscle is attached to the pterygo-mandibular raphe, which is a fibrous band (ligament) extending from the tip of the hamulus to the end of the mylohyoid line. The muscle converges mesially onto the modiolus, where muscle fibres divide and pass into the upper and lower lips.

The buccinator is an accessory muscle of mastication, helping to return the bolus of food from the cheek to the molar teeth for grinding.

Table 3.3 Muscles of mastication

Muscle	Origin	Insertion	Function
Masseter	Maxilla and zygomatic arch	Mandible	Closes jaw
Pterygoids	Pterygoid plates	Mandible	Opens jaw
			Moves jaw laterally
Temporalis	Temporal bone	Coronoid process of mandible	Raises lower jaw
Buccinator	Maxilla and mandible	Obicularis oris	Returns food to teeth
			Pulls corners of mouth laterally

Facial expression

The eyes, nose, and mouth are prominent features of the face. These organs are guarded by the eyelids, nostrils, and lips, respectively. Facial muscles (Fig. 3.7) control these structures and, depending on the functional state of the muscles, various facial expressions are produced as side effects; these muscles are termed 'muscles of facial expression'.

Obicularis oculi

The obicularis oculi muscle has 2 parts: 1 part in the eyelids and 1 going around the eye.

The eyelid part of the muscle closes the eyelids gently and the other part (orbital—around the eye) of the muscle work together to close the eyelids forcibly.

Obicularis oris

The obicularis oris is the muscle that surrounds the opening of the mouth and serves to narrow the mouth to its smallest possible opening (think of pursing your lips!). Some of its fibres come from the buccinators and the others are attached to the mandible and maxilla.

Buccinator

The buccinator contributes to facial expression when the cheeks are puffed out. In this state, the muscle is relaxed; it contracts to expel air from the mouth.

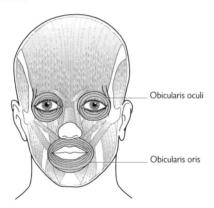

Obicularis oculi

Obicularis oris

Fig. 3.7 Facial muscles.

Tooth development

Deciduous teeth (also known as 'milk teeth' or 'baby teeth') are the first set of teeth to appear in the mouth. These teeth begin to develop during the 6th week of pregnancy and by the 8th week there are 10 areas in both upper and lower jaws that will eventually develop into the deciduous dentition. The teeth begin to calcify (harden) at ~4th month of pregnancy and by the end of the 6th month this process is normally complete. Deciduous teeth begin to erupt (appear) in the mouth at ~5–6 months of age (see Table 3.7). There are 20 teeth in the deciduous dentition, all of which should have erupted by ~2–2.5 years of age.

Eruption of deciduous teeth

Teeth can erupt with little or no problem, but for some babies it can be a long, painful process. There are many different signs and symptoms of teething and these can vary. The more common signs and symptoms are as follows:

- Red and swollen gingiva where the tooth is erupting.
- Flushed cheek or face.
- Rubbing the ear on the same side as the erupting tooth.
- Heavy drooling/dribbling.
- A baby that normally sleeps well might have sleepless nights and stay awake more during the day.
- Inconsistent feeding.
- The child might rub their gingiva in the area where the tooth is appearing or bite/suck items (or anything they can put in their mouth) more often.
- Irritable and unsettled behaviour.

As any parent who has had a child with these signs and symptoms will assure you, teething can be a difficult time! There are various things that can be done to relieve the pain and pressure, such as giving the baby something cold to chew on. Parents should be encouraged to seek advice from their health visitor/doctor for other remedies.

Eruption of permanent teeth

Permanent teeth begin to erupt at ~6 years of age. On average, by the age of 12 years there are no deciduous teeth remaining, because they have all been replaced by permanent teeth. The last of the permanent teeth to erupt are the 3rd molars (also known as 'wisdom teeth'), which normally erupt between 18–25 years of age. Eruption of the permanent dentition does not normally cause as many problems as teething. However, eruption of the 3rd molars can cause a lot of pain and discomfort for adults.

Tooth morphology and function

Tooth morphology is the study of the shape or form of teeth. All teeth have roles; these are outlined here.

Deciduous teeth

Deciduous teeth (Table 3.4) have very white crowns and are often referred to as 'milk teeth' or 'baby teeth'. The dentition comprises 20 teeth: 10 upper and 10 lower teeth. Compared with permanent teeth, deciduous teeth are considerably smaller, the enamel is more prone to wear, the roots are considerably shorter and not as strong, the crowns are more bulbous, and the roots canals are much finer. There are no premolar teeth in the deciduous dentition. All deciduous molars have 4 cusps, except the lower second molar, which has 5.

Permanent teeth

There are 32 teeth in the permanent dentition (Table 3.5): 16 upper and 16 lower teeth. The crowns are off-white in colour. Unlike deciduous teeth, permanent teeth are not replaced once lost. Permanent teeth erupt before the roots have fully formed and the apex is still wide open. It takes ~3 years for the root to be fully formed and the apex to close. The only permanent teeth to erupt with fully formed roots are the canines and the 3rd molars.

Incisors

Permanent incisors have 1 root and a flattened 'chisel-like' crown. The crowns of the upper incisors are much wider than those of the lower incisors. The upper lateral crown is smaller than the upper central crown and the lower central crown is smaller than the lower lateral crown. A small mound in the palatal side of the upper incisors near the cervical margin is called the 'cingulum'. These teeth are used for cutting into food.

Canines

Permanent canines have large, pointed crowns and one long root; the upper canines have the longest roots of all the dentition. The lower canines are smaller than the upper canines. These teeth are also used for cutting into food.

Premolars

Premolars have 2 cusps. The cusps of the upper premolars are almost equal in size but bigger than those of the lower premolars. The lingual cusp of the lower premolars is smaller than the buccal cusp. The upper 1st premolar is the only premolar to have 2 roots; other premolars have 1 root. Premolars are used for chewing.

Molars

Permanent molars have 4 (2 buccal and 2 lingual) cusps, except the lower 1st molar, which has 5 (3 buccal and 2 lingual cusps). Upper 1st molars can often have an additional cusp on the palatal surface, which is called 'the cusp of Caribelli'. Upper molars have 3 roots and lower molars have 2 roots. 3rd molars (wisdom teeth) vary in size and are usually the smallest molars. The number of cusps and roots can vary because the roots are often fused together. Molar teeth are used for chewing food.

Table 3.4 Deciduous teeth

Tooth	Upper roots	Lower roots	Upper cusps	Lower cusps	Function
Central incisor	1	1	Incisal edge	Incisal edge	Cutting
Lateral incisor	1	1	Incisal edge	Incisal edge	Cutting
Canine	1	1	Canine cusp	Canine cusp	Cutting/tearing
First molar	3	2	4	4	Chewing
Second molar	3	2	4	5	Chewing

Table 3.5 Permanent teeth

Tooth	Upper roots	Lower roots	Upper cusps	Lower cusps	Function
Central incisor	1	1	Incisal edge	Incisal edge	Cutting
Lateral incisor	1	1	Incisal edge	Incisal edge	Cutting
Canine	1	1	Canine cusp	Canine cusp	Cutting/tearing
1st premolar	2	1	2	2	Chewing
2nd premolar	1	1	2	2	Chewing
1st molar	3	2	4 and cusp of Caribelli	5	Chewing
2nd molar	3	2	4	4	Chewing
3rd molar	3 (variable)	2 (variable)	4	4	Chewing

Eruption of deciduous teeth

'Eruption' is a term given to the emergence of teeth in the mouth. Deciduous teeth begin erupting ~6 months after birth and this is normally completed by ~24 months of age. The eruption dates of deciduous teeth can vary between individuals, but average dates for eruption are shown in Table 3.6.

The lower deciduous teeth usually erupt before the corresponding upper teeth. Deciduous teeth have a short lifespan and are replaced by permanent teeth. Deciduous teeth become loose by resorption of the roots, which is gradual and begins ~3 years before eruption of the permanent teeth.

Table 3.6 Average eruption dates for deciduous teeth

Tooth	Eruption date
Central incisor	6 months
Lateral incisor	8 months
Canine	18 months
1st molar	12 months
2nd molar	24 months

Eruption of permanent teeth

Permanent teeth begin to erupt in the mouth at ~6 years of age. The first permanent tooth to appear is the 1st molar, which erupts before any of the deciduous teeth have exfoliated (shed) behind the 2nd deciduous molar. Eruption of the permanent dentition is completed with the emergence of the 3rd molars between 18–25 years of age. Similar to the deciduous teeth, the eruption dates for permanent teeth can vary between individuals. The average dates of eruption are shown in Table 3.7 (also see Fig. 3.8).

Unlike the deciduous dentition, the permanent teeth are not replaced once lost. With the exception of the molar teeth, permanent teeth replace deciduous teeth, as outlined in Table 3.8.

Table 3.7 Average eruption dates for permanent teeth

Tooth	Eruption date	
Central incisor	7 years	
Lateral incisor	8 years	
Canine	9 years, lower	11 years, upper
1st premolar	10 years, lower	9 years, upper
2nd premolar	11 years, lower	10 years, upper
1st molar	6 years	
2nd molar	12 years	
3rd molar	18–24 years	

Table 3.8 Replacement of deciduous teeth by permanent teeth

Deciduous tooth	Replacement permanent tooth
Central incisor	Central incisor
Lateral incisor	Lateral incisor
Canine	Canine
1st molar	1st premolar
2nd molar	2nd premolar

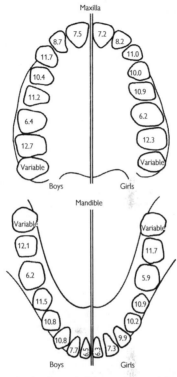

Fig. 3.8 Mean eruption time (in years) of the permanent teeth. Reproduced with permission from Collier J et al. (2009). *Oxford Handbook of Clinical Specialties*, 8th edn. Oxford: OUP.

Tooth structure

Each tooth has a crown, which is the visible part in the mouth, and 1 or more roots, which are hidden inside the jaw. The point at which the crown and root meet is known as 'the neck of the tooth'. The very end of the root is called 'the apex'. Every tooth is made up of enamel, dentine, cementum, and pulp. Enamel, dentine, and cementum are hard, calcified substances and pulp is purely a soft tissue. See Fig. 3.9.

Enamel

Enamel forms the protective outer covering of the crown of the tooth and is translucent in appearance. It is formed by ameloblast cells and made up of 96% inorganic crystals, which are arranged as prisms in an organic matrix. The enamel prisms are long, solid rods that run at right angles to the surface and cemented together by interprismatic substances.

Enamel is the hardest substance in the human body, being harder than bone. Underneath, there is a layer of dentine, which supports the enamel. If this support is lost, the enamel becomes brittle and fractures. Enamel cannot repair itself, so any damage is permanent. Enamel does not contain nerves or blood vessels and ∴ cannot feel any pain.

Dentine

Dentine forms the main bulk of the tooth and resides in the crown and root. Dentine is harder than bone but not as hard as enamel; it is yellowish and gives the tooth its colour. It is formed by ondontoblast cells and is 80% inorganic. The substance is slightly elastic and has a shock-absorbing ability. Unlike enamel, dentine is sensitive to pain, such as extremes of temperature and chemical irritation. It is protected in the crown of the tooth by enamel, which functions as a type of insulation layer. If damaged, dentine can repair itself by producing $2°$ dentine.

Cementum

Cementum covers the dentine in the root of the tooth and has a similar structure to bone. It meets the enamel at the neck of the tooth and varies in thickness in different parts of the tooth. The thickness of the cementum can change, depending on the forces exerted on the teeth.

Pulp

Pulp occupies the centre of the dentine. This soft tissue is made up of nerves and blood vessels and enters the tooth at the root apex. The pulp extends up the root canal into the crown, where it occupies a space called 'the pulp chamber', which is lined by ondontoblast cells.

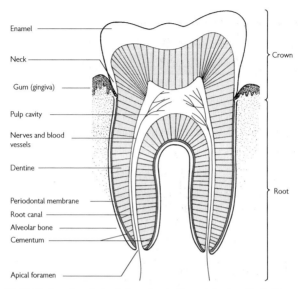

Fig. 3.9 Section of a molar tooth. Reproduced with permission from Martin EA (ed) (2010). *Concise Oxford Medical Dictionary*. Oxford: OUP.

The supporting structures of a tooth

Periodontal ligament

The periodontal ligament is a connective tissue that attaches the tooth to the alveolar bone. The function of the ligament is to ensure that the tooth is attached to the bone, and to support the tooth in the socket.

When pressure is applied to the tooth during chewing and biting, the tooth moves slightly within the socket.

Alveolar bone

Both the mandible and maxilla have a U-shaped dental arch which houses the teeth, this is called the alveolar process. Within the alveolar process, each tooth sits within its own socket known as an alveolar socket. The alveolar ridge is the bony ridge which contains the tooth sockets and the teeth.

Gingiva

The gingiva is the tissue that covers the jaws. Gingival tissue is characterised by a pale pink appearance with stippling. It fits around each tooth like a tight cuff and fills the space in between the teeth to form the interdental papillae.

Nerve supply

The head is supplied by 12 pairs of **cranial nerves**. All of the nerves branch off from the brain, with one from each pair supplying the left side while the other supplies the right side.

The nerves which make muscles and glands work are called **motor nerves** while those that communicate pain and other sensations are called **sensory nerves**.

The cranial nerves that are significant to dental nurses are the **fifth, seventh, ninth** and **twelfth** cranial nerves.

Fifth cranial nerve

This is the most important of all as it supplies the teeth and jaws. It is called the **trigeminal nerve.**

Seventh cranial nerve

This is called the **facial** nerve and supplies the muscles of facial expression. It also provides taste sensory branches to the anterior (front) two-thirds of the **tongue** and motor branches to the **submandibular** and **sublingual** salivary glands.

Ninth cranial nerve

This is known as the **glossopharyngeal nerve.** It supplies sensory branches to the **throat** and the posterior (back) third of the **tongue**. A motor branch of this nerve supplies the parotid gland.

Twelfth cranial nerve

This is called the **hypoglossal nerve** and supplies the muscles of the tongue.

Blood supply

The jaws, teeth, and face are supplied by branches of the **external carotid** artery. Veins draining these parts eventually join the **superior vena cava**.

The **fifth trigeminal nerve** splits in to three divisions: the **ophthalmic, maxillary, and mandibular nerves.** The **maxillary** nerve supplies the upper jaw, its teeth, and the upper part of the face.

The maxillary nerve

See Table 3.9 for a summary of the Maxillary nerves and the teeth and gingiva supplied. The maxillary nerve emerges from the base of the skull and passes forward through the floor of the orbit (Fig. 3.10). Before the maxillary nerve enters the floor of the orbit (eye socket) it branches off to form the **posterior superior alveolar dental nerve** and the **palatine nerves** when the nerve enters the orbit branches to form the **middle superior** and **anterior superior alveolar dental nerve**.

The **posterior superior alveolar** dental nerve enters the back of the maxilla to reach its destination. Once the **anterior superior** and **middle superior alveolar dental nerves** branch off from the maxillary nerve they then pass down inside the maxilla in the walls of the maxillary sinus to reach the teeth (Fig. 3.11).

The **naso palatine nerve** passes through the floor of the nasal cavity to reach the surface of the palate through the **incisive foramen** behind the central incisors.

The **greater palatine nerve** passes through the back of the maxilla and reaches the surface of the hard palate through the **greater palatine foramen** opposite the third molar tooth.

Anterior Superior Alveolar Dental Nerve

This nerve supplies the incisors and canine teeth in the maxilla and the labial gingiva of these teeth.

Middle Superior Alveolar Dental Nerve

The premolars and part of the first molar and the buccal gingiva of these teeth are supplied by this nerve.

Posterior Superior Alveolar Dental Nerve

This nerve supplies the remainder of the first molar, the second and third molars and the buccal gingiva of these teeth.

Naso-palatine nerve

This nerve is also known as the long sphenopalatine nerve. It supplies the palatal gingiva of the incisors and part of the canine.

Greater palatine nerve

This nerve supplies the palatal gingiva of the canine premolars and molars.

Table 3.9 Maxillary nerves and the teeth and gingiva supplied

Nerve	Teeth & gingiva supplied
Anterior superior alveolar dental nerve	Upper central & lateral incisor & canine & labial gingiva
Middle superior alveolar dental nerve	Upper 1st & 2nd Premolar & mesial part of the 1st molar & buccal gingiva
Posterior superior alveolar dental nerve	Distal part of the 1st molar, 2nd & 3rd molar & buccal gingiva
Greater palatine nerve	All palatine gingiva next to the upper molars & premolars, part of the canine
Naso-palatine nerve	All palatine gingiva next to part of the canine, lateral & central incisors

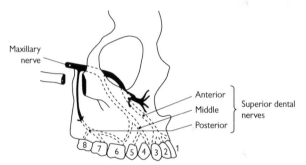

Fig. 3.10 The maxillary nerve and the anatomy of the skull.

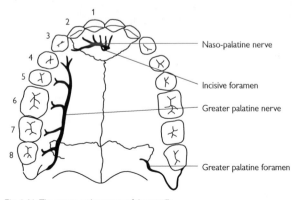

Fig. 3.11 The nerves and anatomy of the maxilla.

The mandibular nerve

See Table 3.10 for a summary of the mandibular nerves and the teeth and gingiva supplied. The maxillary nerve passes down from the base of the skull on the inner side of the ramus of the mandible, between the medial and lateral pterygoid muscles and divides in to branches (Fig. 3.12). The branches are the **inferior dental nerve**, **long buccal nerve**, and the **lingual nerve**.

The **inferior dental nerve** supplies all of the lower teeth and enters the mandible through the **mandibular foramen**. The mandibular foramen can be found at the centre of the inner surface of the mandible and is protected by a bony projection called the **lingula.** After entering the mandibular foramen the inferior dental nerve passes through a canal inside the mandible, the **inferior dental canal**, below the apices of the teeth. Just below the apices of the premolars the nerve branches through the **mental foramen.** Once this branch has emerged through the mental foramen it is referred to as the **mental nerve**.

The **long buccal nerve** passes in to the gingiva on the outer surface of the mandible. The **lingual** nerve passes along the floor of the mouth on the inner surface of the mandible.

Inferior dental nerve

This nerve supplies all of the lower teeth.

Mental nerve

The buccal gingiva of the incisors, canines, premolars, lower lip and chin are all supplied by this nerve.

Long buccal nerve

This nerve supplies the buccal gingiva of the molars.

Lingual nerve

The lingual gingiva of all of the lower teeth is supplied by this nerve.

> **Tip**
>
> Dental nerves e.g. Inferior dental nerve supply teeth and/or gingiva. Nerves, e.g. greater palatine nerve, supply the gingiva.

Table 3.10 Mandibular nerves and the teeth and gingiva supplied

Nerve	Teeth & gingiva supplied
Inferior Dental Nerve	All lower teeth
Mental Nerve	Buccal gingiva of premolar, canine, and incisor teeth
Lingual Nerve	All lingual gingiva
Long Buccal Nerve	Buccal gingiva of molar teeth

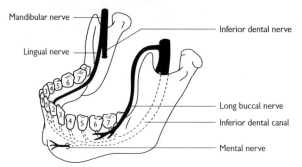

Fig. 3.12 The nerves and anatomy of the lower mandible.

Health and safety

Health and Safety at Work Act 1974

The Health and Safety at Work Act 1974 affects everyone. The Act ensures an individual's health, safety, and welfare at work is protected by law. An employer has a duty of care under the law to protect their employees 'so far as is reasonably practicable' and keep them informed about health and safety issues. 'Reasonably practicable' is a legal term that means allowing the cost of making improvements to be balanced against the benefits. An individual also has a responsibility to look after themselves and others.

What are the employer's legal responsibilities?

- Ensure that the workplace is safe and without risk to health.
- Ensure all machinery, including plant machinery, is safe to use and that safe systems of work are in place and followed.
- Ensure that all substances are used, moved, and stored safely.
- Provide staff with adequate welfare facilities.
- Provide instruction, information training, and supervision necessary for employees' health and safety.

What else must the employer do?

See the Health and Safety Executive's (HSE's) *Health and safety regulation . . . a short guide*:[1]

- Assess risks to health and safety.
- Make arrangements for implementing measures if a risk is identified.
- If the place of work has >5 employees, all findings should be documented in writing.
- Appoint a competent person to assist with health and safety issues.
- Cooperate with other employers if the building is shared.
- Have emergency plans available in the event of an emergency situation.
- Make sure that equipment is only used for its intended use.
- Adequately control or prevent exposure to substances that could be harmful to health.
- Take precautions against flammable or explosive chemicals or materials, including electrical equipment, noise, and radiation.
- Provide health surveillance.
- Avoid hazardous manual-handling operations.
- Provide protective clothing or equipment.
- Ensure safety signs are provided and maintained.

What are the employee's legal responsibilities?

- Take reasonable care of their own health and safety.
- Cooperate with their employer on matters relating to health and safety.
- Correctly use the work equipment provided with by their employer.
- Not to interfere with or misuse equipment provided by their employer.

Further reading

A more detailed analysis of the Health and Safety at Work Act 1974 can be found on the Health and Safety Executive's website: ℘ http://www.hse.gov.uk.

[1] HSE (2003). *Health and safety regulation . . . a short guide*. London: HSE. Available at: ℘ http://www.hse.gov.uk/pubns/hsc13.pdf.

Avoiding hazards in the workplace

Health and safety must be taken seriously. The consequences of accidents at work can be severe. There will always be risks in any workplace, but these can be ↓ by effective standards of health and safety.

Practices to help avoid hazards

- Dental practices benefit from an effective management system that monitors health and safety within the workplace.
- Good communication between all individuals is essential because many issues can be easily resolved.
- All staff should carry out risk assessments, to ↓ the potential for accidents or incidents.
- Safe systems of work should be implemented.
- Good standards of cleaning should be implemented.
- Required maintenance of equipment should be undertaken and recorded at the appropriate intervals.
- All staff, from the cleaner to the principal, should be informed of health and safety matters.
- New staff members require an induction into the practice because working practices vary between establishments.

A member of the dental team or patient might have an accident or incident, but the dental team will be aware of how to deal with the situation if the listed procedures are followed.

Risk assessment

Assessing risk is a legal requirement that should be carried out on an annual basis, unless the risk calls for a more frequent review. Carrying out a risk assessment helps people to think about what could go wrong and look at ways of preventing problems.

Definitions

Hazards

A 'hazard' is anything that has the potential to cause harm, such as:
- Fire.
- Electricity.
- Harmful substances.
- Damaged flooring.

Risks

A 'risk' is the probability that the hazard will cause harm and will depend on many factors. For example, the following should be considered in relation to a damaged floor:
- How bad is the damage?
- How many people walk on the floor?
- Is the area well lit?

A typical assessment

A health and safety risk assessment would typically include the following steps:
- Identification of a hazard.
- Evaluation of the probability that the hazard will occur (risk).
- Deciding who is at risk and in what way.
- Deciding what precautions can be taken to ↓ or eliminate this risk.
- Introducing preventative measures.
- Recording findings and informing colleagues.
- Reviewing the risk assessment periodically and revising it, as necessary.

Risk assessments are usually included in the safety policy document. In an office environment, most assessments can be made on the basis of generic formats.

Specific assessments

Specific assessments must also be made for the following areas, if applicable:
- Visual display equipment.
- Fire.
- Manual handling.

Fire precautions

Fire risk

Once a fire starts, it can spread quickly through a building, producing toxic fumes and smoke. The emphasis is ∴ placed on fire prevention rather than extinguishing a fire.

Fire prevention depends on 3 individual factors, known as 'the fire triangle':

Fuel + Oxygen + Source of ignition = Fire

Fuel

Any material can be classed as 'fuel', but some materials are more hazardous than others. Paper rubbish can easily become hazardous if left to accumulate over a period of time and is sometimes not an obvious hazard. Chemicals, by contrast, can be highly flammable and become a major hazard if they are not kept in a inflammable cupboard.

Oxygen

Oxygen cannot be removed from the atmosphere, but oxygen is depleted by smothering a fire (see 📖 Firefighting, p.71). For a fire to continue, oxygen must be present. Removing the oxygen supply will cause the fire to go out.

Source of ignition

This could be a heat source, such as an electric fire. In certain circumstances the heat source has the potential to ignite, e.g. if it is surrounded by paper.

Evacuation routes

All buildings should have safe exit routes in the event of a fire, such as fire doors and emergency exits. Larger establishments might also have fire-resisting staircases.

Emergency doors must open outwards and should never be locked. If a door is locked, there must be a safe opening system, with clear instructions and an explanation of how to exit the building.

Notices should be clearly displayed and the escape route should be clearly marked. These routes should be checked at all times to ensure that they are not blocked. Fire doors must remain closed at all times and should never be propped open by use of a fire extinguisher.

What to do in the event of a fire?

Everybody in the workplace should be trained in what to do in the event of a fire. Fire drills should be carried out on a regular basis to ensure all staff members are aware of the evacuation procedure. New staff members should be given this information during their induction.

In the event of the fire alarm being sounded, the following should be applied:
- Staff and patients must leave the building immediately by the nearest fire exit.
- If the premises have a lift, this must not be used.
- Staff and patients must not stop to collect personal belongings.
- Staff must close doors behind them.
- Fire wardens, if appointed, should try to sweep through the building and toilets as they leave, so long as this presents no risk.
- Staff and patients must congregate at the designated assembly point— all staff should be aware of this point.
- Staff and patients must not attempt to re-enter the building until the all clear has been given.

Firefighting

❶ It is more important to evacuate a building than attempt to fight a fire and risk becoming trapped. It is dangerous to attempt to tackle a fire if you have no training. In this instance, you should leave the building.

There are many different types of fire extinguisher that can be used, depending on the fire.

Fire extinguishers are generally fixed in suitable locations that are easily accessible, normally in escape routes and by doors. All fire extinguishers should be regularly checked and maintained. New fire extinguishers in the UK are now all coloured 'signal' red to conform to the European Standards. There is an additional coloured strip above the printed instructions on dry powder, foam, and carbon dioxide extinguishers identifying their contents (Table 4.1).

Table 4.1 Fire extinguisher colour codes and uses

Contents	Water	Powder	Foam	Carbon dioxide
Coloured strip code	None	Blue	Cream	Black
Can be used on	• Paper • Wood • Textiles • Solid materials	• Liquid • Electrical • Paper • Textiles	• Liquid • Paper • Wood • Textiles	• Liquid • Electrical
Not to be used on	• Liquid • Electrical • Metals	• Metal	• Electrical • Metal	• Metal

Control of Substances Hazardous to Health (COSHH) Regulations

Workplace exposure

Using chemicals or other hazardous substances at work can put an individual's health at risk. The dental surgery uses many chemicals, ranging from disinfectants to developing solutions. The law 6 requires employers to control exposure to hazardous substances, preventing ill health. There are 8 basic steps that should be followed:

- Assess the risk.
- Decide what precautions are needed.
- Prevent or adequately control exposure.
- Ensure that control measures are used and maintained.
- Monitor the exposure.
- Carry out the appropriate health surveillance.
- Prepare plans and procedures to deal with accidents, incidents, and emergencies.
- Ensure employees are properly informed, trained, and supervised.

Which substances are covered by the regulations?

COSHH Regulations apply to virtually all substances hazardous to health, with the following exceptions:

- Asbestos and lead—which have their own regulations.
- Biological agents—which are outside the employer's control (e.g. catching a cold from a workmate).

Working with hazardous substances

These regulations are there for the safety of all individuals. Before using any substance, whether it is a liquid, powder, spray cream, or an aerosol, take the following steps:

- Identify whether the substance is hazardous by either reading the enclosed instruction leaflet or checking the container for a hazard symbol, which would be on the side of the container.
- If there is a hazard symbol on the container, go to the COSHH file.
- Look up the procedures you must take when using the substance.
- Follow the recommended protection procedures.
- If you have an accident, refer to the hazard safety data sheet.
- If you have any concerns, refer to the manufacturer.

Reporting of Injuries, Diseases, and Dangerous Occurrences Regulations (RIDDOR)

All workplaces are required by law to report accidents that cause major injuries or dangerous occurrences. An accident/incident book should be kept in the dental practice and all employees should be aware of its location. The best location for the book would be in an administrative area, such as the reception, to which all employees have access.

Examples of major injuries

- Fracture of the skull, spine, or pelvis.
- Fracture of the long bones in the arm or leg.
- Amputation of the hand or foot.
- Loss of sight in eyes.
- Hypoxia severe enough to produce unconsciousness.
- Any other injury that requires the patient to stay in hospital for >24 hours.

Examples of dangerous occurrences

- Explosion.
- Collapse of an autoclave or compressor.
- An uncontrolled release of mercury vapour—normally as a result of a major mercury spillage.
- Any case of acute ill health owing to pathogens or infectious material.

▶ It is essential that both staff members and patients are aware of what should be reported. That is, all accidents that occur on the premises, no matter how trivial, should be reported, in addition to the examples listed here. This includes violent assaults or attacks that happen in the practice, which should also be reported to the police.

Hazardous Waste Regulations

What is hazardous waste?

Hazardous waste is discarded material that can pose a substantial risk to the health of the general public health or environment. Hazardous waste should be disposed of using the methods appropriate to the particular type of waste (see 📖 Waste disposal and the Environmental Protection Act, p.76).

❶ Placing clinical waste into black refuse sacks is inappropriate and should not be done under any circumstances.

The Hazardous Waste Regulations ensure that the following processes are carried out:

- Identification of hazardous waste.
- Ensure safe management of hazardous waste at all times.
- Provide written documentation for the movement of hazardous waste, from the site of origin to the final disposal point.
- Require people who receive hazardous waste to keep thorough records.

Clinical waste

Clinical waste is defined in regulation 1(2) of The Controlled Waste Regulations 1992 (SI1992/588) as:

(a) any waste which consists wholly or partly of human or animal tissue, blood, other body fluids, excretion, drugs or other pharmaceutical products, swabs or dressings, or syringes, needles or other sharp instruments, being waste which unless rendered safe may prove hazardous to any person coming into contact with it; and

(b) any other waste arising from medical, nursing, dental, veterinary, pharmaceutical or similar practice, investigation treatment, care, teaching or research, or the collection of blood for transfusion, being waste which may cause infection to any person coming into contact with it.

The dental surgery has the means to produce a significant volume of clinical waste on a daily basis, including the following:

- Sharps.
- Amalgam.
- Spent fixing and developing chemicals.

All these materials require special disposal. Dental nurses must be aware of the disposal methods of each material and ensure that the appropriate procedure is carried out at all times.

Non-clinical waste

Non-clinical waste, such as paper and boxes, can be disposed of with general waste or recycled.

Waste containing personal details

Any material containing patients' personal information should be shredded, ensuring confidentiality is maintained.

Working with hazardous and non-hazardous waste

The dental nurse should take precautions to prevent injury and cross-infection when working with both hazardous and non-hazardous waste.

Protective equipment

- Disposable gloves and safety spectacles should always be worn when handling waste in the dental surgery.
- A mask should also be worn to prevent inhalation when handling waste chemicals or substances that emit harmful vapours, such as mercury.

Sharps boxes

- The dental nurse should ensure that waste is placed into the correct containers and appropriate places for storage and collection.
- Care should be taken when locking sharps boxes and under no circumstances should the dental nurse place their hands or fingers inside.
- The contents of a sharps bin can be levelled by gently shaking the container from side to side, to dislodge any items that might be protruding.

In case of sharps injury, see 📖 Bleeding: cuts and grazes, p.122.

Records of hazardous waste disposal

Records of collection of all types of waste should be kept and signed by both the collection company and the dental surgery. Records related to non-sharps and sharps clinical waste should be kept for 2 years and those related to special waste should be kept for 3 years.

Waste disposal and the Environmental Protection Act

As a dental nurse, you must know how to correctly dispose of a variety of different forms of waste in the dental surgery. With so many forms of waste in the surgery, the dental nurse can easily become confused.

Non-sharps clinical waste

Examples
- Cotton wool rolls.
- Gauze.
- Tissue.

Disposal
- Dispose of non-sharps clinical waste in a yellow or orange clinical waste bag (marked in black as 'hazardous waste'), which are collected by an authorized disposal contractor.
- When bags are 3/4 full, the air should be expelled and the bags securely tied at the neck.
- Bags should be stored to prevent unauthorized access.

Most clinical waste companies supply the dental practice with the bags and a lockable container to store filled bags before collection. After collection, the waste is incinerated. Legislation is complex and changes; a reputable company will comply with current regulations.

Sharps clinical waste

Examples
- Needles.
- Scalpel blades.
- Objects that might puncture a clinical waste bag.

Disposal
- Sharps clinical waste must be disposed of (ideally by the dentist) in plastic, lockable, rigid, puncture-proof containers and collected by an authorized disposal contactor.
- Sharps containers are supplied by waste disposal companies and should be no more than 3/4 full.
- Ensure sharps boxes are constructed correctly and, while in use, stored so that unauthorized access is prevented. For example, a bright yellow sharps box can be tempting for a young child.
- When 3/4 full, sharps bins should be locked and placed in a secure location for collection for incineration.
- Containers should be dated and labelled so they can be traced back to their source.

Chemicals

Examples
- Developer and fixer used in developing radiographs.

Disposal
- Chemicals must not be disposed of down the sink because they are harmful to the environment.
- After use, the solutions should be placed in a secure, plastic screw-top container (supplied by the waste collection contractor), to await collection.

Special waste

Drugs

Drugs left over, such as local anaesthetic cartridges that are not completely empty or out-of-date drugs, should be disposed of separately.

These agents are placed into a rigid, puncture-proof, lockable, container that is collected by an authorized contactor. These containers should only be 3/4 full, then locked and kept securely until collection.

Other special waste

Amalgam, amalgam capsules and sundries, and extracted teeth have their own separate containers for disposal. These are rigid, screw-top containers that are also collected by authorized waste contractors. Containers used for amalgam have a special sponge inside that has been soaked in potassium permanganate to help absorb mercury and mercury vapours.

▶ The Environmental Protection Act

The aim of the Environmental Protection Act is to prevent air, land, or water becoming polluted by emissions. Similar to most legislation, it places a duty of care on each individual to ensure that waste is disposed of appropriately. This will include those producing the waste, those contracted to collect the waste, and those disposing of the waste.

An example of when you could be held responsible by this Act is the inappropriate disposal of chemicals related to fixing and developing solutions. Unless permission is sought from the local water authority, spent chemicals should not be tipped down the sink. If in doubt, the manufacturers should be consulted and adequate instructions obtained. When these instructions arrive, they should be read and fully understood before carrying out any disposal.

Infection control

Micro-organisms

Many diseases are caused by micro-organisms, but not all micro-organisms are harmful. Those that are harmful to the human body are known as pathogenic (more commonly called 'germs') and those that are not harmful are non-pathogenic.

There are 3 main groups to be aware of in the dental surgery: bacteria, viruses, and fungi.

Bacteria

Bacterial infections can be treated by using antibacterial drugs such as antibiotics (see 📖 Antibacterial agents, p.346). Bacterial infections can be classed as aerobic or anaerobic, according to the type of bacteria present.

Aerobic bacteria require oxygen to survive, whilst anaerobic bacteria are able to survive in areas without oxygen.

Bacteria can be classified according to their shape:

Cocci (round bacteria)
- Staphylococci grow in clumps and are responsible for skin and gum boils.
- Streptococci grow in single strands, and one species (*Streptococcus mutans*) is responsible for beginning the caries process.

Bacilli (rod shaped)
- Lactobacilli can be found in decayed teeth.
- *Bacillus fusiformis* can be found in acute ulcerative gingivitis (AUG).

Spirochaetes (spiral shaped)
These can also be found in AUG in the form of *Borrelia vincentii*.

Bacterial spores
Some bacteria can survive unfavourable conditions (such as extremes of temperature and drought) in the form of spores. They form a tough outer coating around themselves and can lie dormant for years. When conditions become favourable they can resume their active state. Spores are highly resistant to destruction and a special method of sterilization is required to destroy them.

Viruses

Theses are much smaller than bacteria and need a special microscope (electron microscope) to be viewed.

Viruses cause a variety of diseases including influenza, herpes, hepatitis B, human immunodeficiency virus (HIV), and rabies. Treating a viral infection is very difficult. Antibiotics do not have any effect on viruses, and few antiviral drugs are known.

Fungi

Fungi are the largest micro-organisms, and infections can be treated using antifungal drugs (see 📖 Antifungal agents, p.352). The most significant fungus found in the mouth is *Candida albicans,* which causes denture stomatitis and thrush. Denture stomatitis—also known as 'denture sore mouth'—appears as red areas underneath dentures or removable appliances. Thrush, which appears as white patches in the mouth and on the tongue, is most commonly found in babies or in the mouths of run-down elderly people.

Other significant infective agents

Prions are a type of infectious agent made up only of proteins. They cause a number of diseases in animals including bovine spongiform encephalopathy (BSE) in cattle, and Creutzfeldt–Jakob disease (CJD) in humans (see ⛶ Creutzfeldt–Jakob disease (CJD), p.88). Prion diseases affect the brain or other neural tissue, and are all currently untreatable and fatal.

Prions cannot be removed by normal sterilization procedures, and your practice policy should be followed before, during, and after treatment for patients with prion diseases.

Hepatitis B

Hepatitis B is an inflammation of the liver caused by the hepatitis B virus. The hepatitis B virus represents a significant risk to dental personnel, as it can be transferred via the instruments that are used on a day-to-day basis. When a person is first infected with the hepatitis B virus, it is commonly known as an acute infection. A majority of adults will fight off the virus, developing antibodies in the process, thus ensuring that the body can protect itself if they become exposed again.

For those who still have the virus present in their blood after 6 months it is assumed that the virus will stay in the blood and liver for the lifetime of the person. This is known as chronic hepatitis. Most people with chronic hepatitis live long and healthy lives; however, there is an ↑ chance that they can develop serious liver disease in the future. A chronic infection relating to hepatitis B can lead to cirrhosis. This is a condition where the cells of the liver are scarred by tissue fibres. This in turn can cause the liver to become less effective and over time leads to liver failure.

Transmission

Hepatitis B is transmitted in several different ways. These include unprotected sexual intercourse, blood transfusions (prior to more rigid screening programmes introduced in 1992), blood-to-blood contact, use of contaminated needles and syringes, body piercing, tattooing (if needles not sterile), and vertical transmission from mother to baby during childbirth. In the dental surgery the virus can be contracted via a puncture wound from a contaminated instrument or needle.

Symptoms

Symptoms will vary in each patient; however, these can be confused with flu-like symptoms such as abdominal pain, loss of appetite, nausea and vomiting, and joint pain. More severe symptoms include yellowing of the eyes and skin (otherwise known as jaundice), and a bloated or swollen stomach.

Treatment

For acute hepatitis B no treatment is necessary other than careful monitoring of liver and other body functions with blood tests. For chronic hepatitis B there is a wide range of drugs available, which will help slow the virus. These would be prescribed on an individual basis.

Prevention

All clinical members of the dental team who have direct contact with patients undergoing dental treatment should be vaccinated against hepatitis B. Once a course has been completed immunity levels will need to be checked every 5–10 years depending on the individual. Within the dental surgery, methods of reducing injuries can be adopted. This may include the use of safety syringes, which ↓ the risk of needlestick injuries. Care should also be taken when cleaning instruments prior to sterilization.

Hepatitis C

Hepatitis C is an inflammation of the liver caused by the hepatitis C virus. The virus represents a significant risk to dental personnel. Again, this is related to the instruments that we use on a day-to-day basis.

Transmission

Hepatitis C is transmitted by blood-to-blood contact. This can be through blood transfusions (prior to more rigid screening programmes introduced in 1992), the use of contaminated needles and syringes through drug abuse, through needles during body piercing, and tattooing (if needles not sterile). In the dental surgery, the virus can be contracted via a puncture wound from a contaminated instrument or needle.

Symptoms

Many patients who contract hepatitis C have no symptoms and are unaware that they are carrying the virus. In the handful of people who do develop symptoms these can be confused with flu-like symptoms, such as fatigue and a loss of appetite. This means that the virus is not normally detected until the patient has a routine blood test or visits a GP for some other reason. It is not until the virus develops further that more telltale signs develop due to the liver becoming compromised. Possible indications of the advanced virus include: bruising for no reason, a tendency to bleed more, pain in the bones, enlarged veins and jaundice. Should these symptoms develop, then further investigation should be carried out.

Treatment

The aim of hepatitis C medication is control of liver disease symptoms, improvement of liver function, prevention of cirrhosis of the liver and liver cancer, and, optimally, to cure.

Prevention

At present there is no vaccination against hepatitis C. As with all blood-borne transmissible diseases care should be taken when handling a majority of dental instruments. This may include the use of safety syringes, which ↓ the risk of needlestick injuries. Care should be taken when cleaning instruments prior to sterilization.

Hepatitis: other forms

Table 5.1 Other forms of hepatitis

Hepatitis	Notes	Prevention	Transmission	Symptoms	Treatment
A	Does not normally have a chronic phase; does not normally lead to any permanent damage	Vaccine protects for 15–30 years; improving sanitation; improving personal hygiene; personal towels and toothbrushes for the individual	Faecal–oral; easily spread where sanitation and personal hygiene are poor	Can be mistaken for flu. Appears 2–6 weeks after infection. Fatigue; fever; abdominal pains; nausea; diarrhoea; loss of appetite; jaundice	Rest, avoid fatty foods, and eat a well-balanced diet
D	Can only replicate in individuals who already have hepatitis B	Those at risk of contracting hepatitis B should be vaccinated. Those who have contracted hepatitis B should be educated, to reduce risk of transmission	Unprotected sex; blood transfusions; blood-to-blood contact; contaminated needles and syringes; body piercing; tattooing; transmission from mother to baby during childbirth	Jaundice; fatigue; abdominal pain; loss of appetite; nausea; vomiting; joint pain; dark coloured urine	Hepatitis B vaccine given to prevent hepatitis B/D virus co-infection

E	Endemic in Asia, Africa, and the Middle East, where water quality can be poor. More severe in pregnant women, especially in the 3rd trimester	Clean water supplies and hygienic practices. Hand washing with soap and water after using the bathroom and when preparing food. Drinking water should be avoided if the source is unknown.	Faeco-oral; can be passed from person-to-person or from a zoonotic (animal) host	Jaundice; fatigue; abdominal pain; loss of appetite; nausea, vomiting; joint pain; dark coloured urine	No specific treatment
G	Discovered more recently. Little is known about it, though it appears to be related to hepatitis C	Relies on avoiding contact with blood	Transmission of hepatitis G closely follows that of hepatitis B and C	Currently unspecified	No specific treatment; rest, avoid alcohol, and eat a well-balanced diet

Methicillin-resistant *Staphylococcus aureus* (MRSA)

This strain of bacterium is from the *Staphylococcus aureus* species. It is estimated that 1 in 3 people carry the bacteria on their skin/nostrils but do not develop an infection. Nevertheless should the bacteria be able to enter the body it can cause infections in different parts of the body, resulting in boils, abscesses, or impetigo. Should the bacterium reach the bloodstream, more serious infections can occur.

Whilst MRSA is no more infectious than other forms of *Staph. aureus*, it is difficult to treat as it has become resistant to many forms of antibiotics including penicillin, forms of methicillin, and cephalosporins.

Transmission

As *Staph. aureus* bacteria live on the skin they are easily spread by direct skin contact. This is often via people's hands. This is one reason why strict hand-hygiene measures are so important. MRSA is also spread via bedding, towels, clothing, and equipment.

Symptoms

The symptoms of MRSA infection depend on where the person has been infected.

MRSA most often appears as a skin infection, like a boil or abscess. It also might infect a surgical wound. In either case, the area would look:
• Swollen.
• Red.
• Painful.
• Pus filled.

If MRSA infects the lungs and causes pneumonia, the person might have:
• Shortness of breath.
• Fever.
• Chills.

Treatment

MRSA is difficult to treat with antibiotics. Each case will be evaluated and the appropriate antibiotic and dose will be given.

Vancomycin-resistant *Staphylococcus aureus* (VRSA)

VRSA is a strain of *Staph. aureus* that has become resistant to the antibiotic vancomycin. This has made VRSA more difficult to treat. Each case should be managed by the appropriate medical practitioner.

Human immunodeficiency virus (HIV)

HIV is a virus responsible for targeting and destroying the cells in our immune systems that help us fight off infections. CD4 cells are a type of white blood cell which help to protect the body from illness and also coordinate various activities of the immune system.

HIV attacks CD4 cells, before replicating within the body. As the CD4 cells are depleted, the immune system becomes weaker and the body is less able to fight infections.

A normal CD4 cell count is about 600–1500 cells per cubic millimetre of blood. The CD4 cell count usually drops as HIV progresses.

Transmission

HIV is normally only spread through blood, semen, vaginal fluids and breast milk. The most common ways of contracting HIV are:

- By re-using and sharing needles, especially common in drug users.
- Unprotected sexual intercourse.
- Mother-to-child transmission during pregnancy, birth, and breastfeeding.

In dentistry, the primary concern relates to injuries obtained via needles or sharp instruments within the dental surgery.

Signs and symptoms

It can take up to 12 weeks for HIV to be detected in the body and for a test to come back positive. However, flu-like symptoms may occur 2–4 weeks after exposure. These can include swollen glands, fever, muscle aches, and a rash.

Treatment

There is currently no known cure for HIV. Antiviral drugs can help improve the quality of life for those who are HIV-positive, and help them to stay healthier for longer, but this is not a cure. Once medication is started, the patient should see a reduction in the viral load (the amount of virus in the blood). The viral load is determined by a blood test.

Despite receiving antiviral medication, a patient may start to see their viral load ↑ (more virus in the blood) at some stage. This can be due to the virus' ↑ 'resistance'. A virus is referred to as being 'resistant' to a particular drug when the action of that drug becomes less effective. This then means that the patient's treatment regimen will need to be reviewed.

Prevention

Within the dental surgery there should be a safe system in use to remove and dispose of sharps. Safety syringes are now available which provide protection against injury if used in accordance with the manufacturers' instructions. Blade removers are also available. Particular care and attention should be paid to smaller sharps, such as suture needles, which can easily become lost on a surgical tray.

Creutzfeldt–Jakob disease (CJD)

CJD is a degenerative and usually fatal brain disorder caused by a type of infectious protein called a prion (see ☐ Other significant infective agents p.81). Symptoms may include dementia, problems with muscular movements and coordination, impaired vision and memory. As the patient's condition deteriorates, they can also suffer from depression and insomnia.

It is thought that CJD can not be transmitted through the air, by touching people, or by other forms of contact; however, the exact transmission route/s is unclear.

At present there is no treatment for CJD and it is not normally diagnosed until a postmortem is carried out.

CJD is a rare condition that is seldom encountered by the dental profession; however it is imperative that the dental team recognize that normal sterilization methods used in the general surgery would have no effect on the prion protein.

Herpes simplex

Herpes simplex is a viral infection. The most common form of herpes simplex that dental nurses will see is the type 1 virus. Herpes simplex type 2 is less significant in relation to dentistry (as it is most commonly associated with genital infections) but you should be aware of the virus as it can also be oral.

Transmission

In the case of herpes simplex type 1, it is transmitted by kissing or other close contact with an individual. The virus can lay dormant in the nerve endings until it is triggered by factors such as fever, exposure to the sun, feeling run down, and during menstruation. Many infected people do not even know that they are infected.

Signs and symptoms

Sometimes the patient will complain about itching and burning around the infected area. This is then followed by the appearance of a small group of red blisters, commonly on the lips. After a few days the blisters begin to dry up and form a crust over the top. This in time will fall off and the redness ↓. Some people have no symptoms at all.

Treatment

There is a wide selection of treatments available for herpes. These can either be taken by mouth or applied direct to the infected area. However, they only shorten an outbreak. They do not prevent outbreaks from happening.

Prevention

Herpes is very difficult to prevent as so many people may already have the virus. However, things can be done to help. Family members should not share towels or linen with anyone who has an active outbreak. The person with the attack should maintain good hand hygiene to avoid spreading the virus.

Should a patient phone or come in to the dental surgery with an outbreak, care should be taken about treating the patient due to the nature of transmission. In some cases it may be best to cancel the patient's appointment. This of course will be at the dentist's discretion.

Childhood diseases

Children come into contact with all sorts of infections and illnesses. If a child is ill it is advisable to cancel the appointment until the child recovers. Common illnesses include measles, mumps, rubella, chickenpox, and whooping cough. It is essential that all dental nurses are vaccinated against the common childhood illnesses as well as polio, TB, and hepatitis B.

Measles

Measles is a highly contagious viral infection. It can cause a rash which can cover the whole body. The child can also complain of flu-like symptoms which will include a temperature, cough, and a runny nose. Measles is transmitted when a child sneezes or coughs. The virus is spread through droplets which travel in the air.

Mumps

Mumps is another viral infection which is spread through saliva and can infect many parts of the body, especially the parotid salivary glands. In cases of mumps these glands start to swell and become very painful.

Rubella

Rubella or German measles as it is also known is another of the viral infections. It is caused by the rubella virus which is not the same virus as that of measles. Again it can be transmitted from droplets from the nose or throat which others in close proximity inhale.

Chickenpox

Chickenpox is a common virus among children and is caused by the varicella zoster virus. Unfortunately this virus can lie dormant in the body. A child normally only has one bout of chickenpox, nevertheless in adults due to its dormant tendencies it can emerge as shingles.

Whooping cough

Whooping cough, or pertussis as it can also be known, is a bacterial infection. The patient will have a severe coughing fit. At the end of the fit as the patient breaths in a 'whooping' sound may be heard; hence the name whooping cough. Transmission is through respiratory secretions spread during coughing and sneezing.

Tuberculosis (TB)

TB is a disease caused by the bacteria *Mycobacterium tuberculosis*. This bacterium mainly affects the lungs. However, it can also attack other parts of the human body such as the spine, brain, and kidneys. If not treated, this can prove to be fatal.

Transmission

TB is transmitted in the air; thus it is an airborne disease. Bacteria are released into the air when an infected person coughs or sneezes. People in the surrounding area may breathe in the bacteria and become infected themselves. The bacteria can settle in the lungs and begin to grow and from here it can move around the body. It is most likely to be transmitted to those individuals who live with the infected person.

Signs and symptoms

Signs and symptoms may include a cough lasting for >3 weeks, unexplained weight loss, fatigue, ↑ temperature, night sweats, a loss of appetite, and sometimes pain on breathing and coughing.

Treatment

Treatment for TB is normally through antibiotic medication prescribed by the GP who will be looking after the patient.

Prevention

Patients should always take any medication that has been prescribed by the GP and should always cover their mouth with a tissue when coughing, sneezing, or laughing. The tissue should then be placed in a closed bag and thrown away. Children should not go to school or adults to work. Sleep in a *separate* bedroom away from other family members to avoid transmission. Patients with TB should not attend the dental surgery and all appointments should be cancelled until fully fit.

Cross infection and transmission

Cross infection can be defined as: infection which is transmitted from one person to another in the dental surgery, during treatment procedures, or in the waiting room by inadequately sterilized instruments, materials, or equipment.

Infection can be spread from:
• Patient to patient.
• Patient to dental team.
• Dental team to patient.
• Dental team to dental team.

Routes of transmission

Direct

Direct transmission of infection takes place when one person infects another by direct person-to-person contact (e.g. shaking hands). Hands are the source of transmission of infectious particles from patient to patient, if adequate hand washing practices are not enforced (see Fig. 5.1).

Several people in the practice can become infected in this way, including the clinician, dental nurse, receptionist, patient, dental technician, and any cleaning staff.

Indirect

Contact results in the transmission of infectious particles from person to person via a carrier. Objects such as eating utensils, medical instruments, or equipment used in food preparation may become contaminated with a pathogenic micro-organism and in turn spread the disease to other individuals. Infected needles may also be the source of indirect transmission of pathogens between people.

Inhalation

Airborne droplets which are expelled by an infected individual by sneezing or coughing can be inhaled by another individual in close proximity. Expelled droplets may travel for several metres before falling and therefore are easily spread to surrounding individuals. An example of diseases caused by the inhalation of infectious droplets includes influenza (or 'flu', caused by the influenza virus).

Inoculation

An inoculation injury—or sharps injury—occurs when an instrument (typically a needle contaminated with blood) punctures the skin.

For any member of the dental team, this can be one of the most worrying injures that is sustained.

This provides a direct transmission route into the bloodstream. In the event of a suspected inoculation transmission, the practice should follow their local policy.

Ingestion
Transmission can occur when pathogenic organisms are ingested and then enter the gastrointestinal tract. This typically occurs when the organisms are excreted by an infected person, and are then carried on the hands or via food. This is therefore called the 'faecal–oral' route. This is apparent in the transmission of hepatitis A. Due to the nature of the transmission this is the most unlikely to occur in the dental surgery.

Methods of infection control

Universal precautions

The procedures/methods listed in Table 5.2 can be used to control the spread of infection in the dental surgery:

Table 5.2 Precautions against infection

Disposables	Single-use, disposable items such as aspirator tips, barrier shields, gloves, 3 in 1 tips should be used wherever possible
Zoning	The dental surgery should be divided into different areas of use. Areas should be identified for contaminated and non-contaminated instruments, materials, and equipment to reduce the risk of cross infection
Personal protective equipment (PPE)	This should be worn during all clinical procedures, when preparing for and clearing away following dental procedures, preparing instruments for sterilization and when handling chemicals (see ☐ Personal protective equipment (PPE), p.96)
Ultrasonic cleaning	All instruments with the exception of dental hand pieces should be placed in an ultrasonic bath prior to sterilization to remove debris. The solution in the bath should be made up following the manufacturers' recommended instructions
Sterilization	All dental instruments that are not single use, should be sterilized adequately before use (see ☐ Principles of sterilization, p.100)
Disinfection	Disinfection of all dental surfaces and equipment should be carried out before and after each patient. Items sent to and from the lab, e.g. impressions, wax rims, should also be disinfected (see ☐ Disinfection, p.101)
Effective hand cleansing	• Minimal jewellery should be worn • Nails kept short with no polish • All cuts and abrasions should be covered with a waterproof dressing • Hands moisturized daily • Hands should be washed using the correct procedure at the beginning of every treatment session • A disinfectant hand rub can be used in between patients (see ☐ Hand hygiene, p.98)
Waste disposal	Waste should be disposed of in the correct manner, in the correct waste disposal containers
Vaccination	All of the dental team should have the following vaccinations: • MMR (measles, mumps & rubella) • Poliomyelitis • Tetanus • Pertussis • Diphtheria • TB • Hepatitis B

Table 5.2 (Contd.)

Up-to-date medical history	Every patient should have their medical history updated at every visit for both the protection of the patient and the dental team. For example, staff will be made aware if the patient has a disease that could be transmitted and also be aware if the patient is immunocompromised and may be more susceptible to infection
Good personal hygiene	All members of the dental team should maintain good standards of personal hygiene at all times

Asepsis

Aseptic techniques attempt to eliminate or reduce pathogenic micro-organisms entering the clinical working area.

Aseptic techniques

Where there is a possibility of introducing pathogenic micro-organisms into the body a 'no touch' technique is used. Every instrument used must be sterile (not just surgically clean) and must be handled and stored in a manner to prevent contamination.

Following the appropriate infection control procedures in the clinical area will help maintain an aseptic technique and prevent infection.

Personal protective equipment (PPE)

PPE should be available for both staff and patients to wear in the clinical environment.

Clothing/footwear

A clinical uniform/clothing should be worn when working in the clinical environment. This should not be worn when travelling to and from a place of work and should be changed every day. Uniforms/clothing should be laundered at a minimum temperature of 65°C, following the manufacturer's instructions. Closed-toed footwear should be worn and ideally be leather lace-ups with rubber soles. The practice policy should be followed at all times with regards to uniform regulations.

Disposable gloves/heavy duty gloves

Disposable gloves should only be worn in the clinical environment and should be worn during all clinical procedures, when disinfecting the clinical bay, and when handling chemicals. Gloves should be discarded after use or when they become damaged or heavily soiled. Latex-free gloves are available for staff and patients with latex allergies.

Heavy duty gloves should be worn when handling/preparing instruments prior to sterilization.

Disposable masks

Masks should only be worn in the clinical environment and should be worn during all clinical procedures and when preparing instruments for sterilization. Masks should also be worn when there is any risk of inhalation or ingestion of substances such as chemicals.

Eye protection

Safety glasses or visors should only be worn in the clinical environment and should be worn during all clinical procedures and when preparing instruments for sterilization. Eye protection should be worn by both the dental team and the patient to prevent any debris, blood/body fluids, chemicals, or infected materials entering the eyes.

Disposable aprons

Disposable aprons can be worn when soiling may occur in dental and cleaning procedures. These help to protect the uniform and skin FRM splashes from blood/saliva, chemicals, and infected materials.

Bibs/napkins

Disposable bibs/napkins should be worn by the patient during all clinical procedures to protect their clothes from contamination from dental materials and blood/saliva.

Hand hygiene

One of the most effective methods of preventing the spread of infection in the clinical environment is good hand hygiene.

Preventing micro-organism build-up

To reduce the areas where micro-organisms can accumulate on the hands:
- Nails should be kept short with no nail polish.
- Wounds should be covered with a waterproof dressing.
- Minimal jewellery (rings, watches, bracelets) should be worn.
- Hands should be moisturized to prevent dry skin and cracking.

Washing

Before every clinical session hands should be washed effectively using the following technique:
- Remove all jewellery and roll up sleeves.
- Turn on the tap using the foot or elbow control.
- Wet hands and apply a liquid soap such as HiBiscrub® from a elbow-operated dispenser.
- Clean all surfaces of the hands including the wrists (see Fig. 5.1).
- Rinse hands thoroughly under running water, holding the hands downwards.
- Turn off the tap using the foot or elbow control.
- Dry hands thoroughly with disposable paper towel.

To protect hands further, ensure that disposable gloves are worn during every clinical procedure, when handling chemicals, and when preparing the clinical area. Wear heavy duty gloves when preparing contaminated instruments for sterilization.

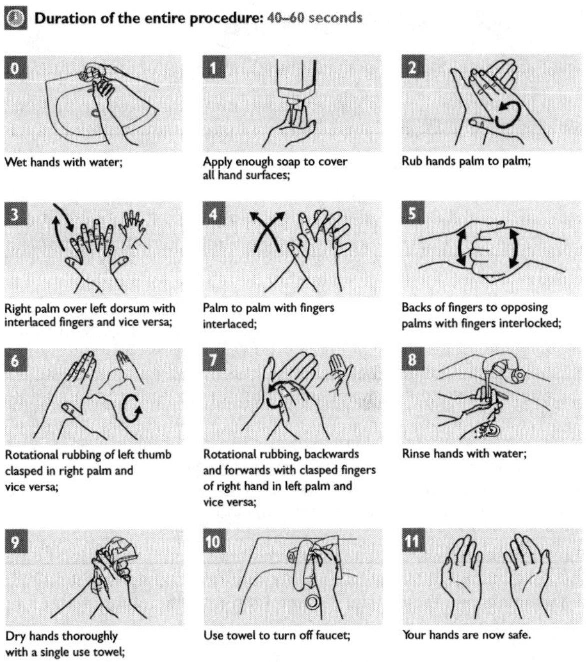

Duration of the entire procedure: 40–60 seconds

0	**1**	**2**
Wet hands with water;	Apply enough soap to cover all hand surfaces;	Rub hands palm to palm;
3	**4**	**5**
Right palm over left dorsum with interlaced fingers and vice versa;	Palm to palm with fingers interlaced;	Backs of fingers to opposing palms with fingers interlocked;
6	**7**	**8**
Rotational rubbing of left thumb clasped in right palm and vice versa;	Rotational rubbing, backwards and forwards with clasped fingers of right hand in left palm and vice versa;	Rinse hands with water;
9	**10**	**11**
Dry hands thoroughly with a single use towel;	Use towel to turn off faucet;	Your hands are now safe.

Fig. 5.1 Hand washing procedure. Reproduced with permission from WHO guidelines on hand hygiene in health care (2009).

Principles of sterilization

Sterilization kills bacteria, spores, fungi, and viruses and is the most effective method of preventing cross infection in the dental surgery. As different materials are used to make the various items of dental instruments, there are different methods of sterilization to suit.

Autoclave sterilization

An autoclave produces steam under pressure which has the ability to kill bacteria, spores, fungi, and viruses. It is suitable for metal instruments and burs, rubber, most plastics, cotton wool, and paper points. Before instruments can be placed in the autoclave they must (with the exception of dental hand pieces) first be placed in the ultrasonic bath. Wearing safety specs and heavy duty gloves the instruments should be scrubbed under running water with a stiff brush. They should be placed into the bath for the duration specified by the manufacturer. Once the cycles complete they should be removed, rinsed under running water, and placed into the autoclave. Hand pieces should be wiped to remove debris and oiled prior to sterilization. Some instruments are placed into special sterilization pouches to help maintain sterility. All instruments should be evenly spaced in open trays to make sure all surfaces are exposed during the cycle. The manufacturer's instructions should be followed when using the autoclave. Once the cycle begins the autoclave produces steam up to a pressure of 2.2 bars and a temperature of 134°C. The contents are held at this temperature and pressure for a minimum of 3 minutes to gain sterility and then are cooled down. The full cycle should take approximately 15–20 minutes. Once instruments are sufficiently cooled they can be removed and stored appropriately.

Autoclaves

There are three types of autoclave:

Type N

These are non-vacuum autoclaves and are suitable for non-wrapped instruments.

Type B

These are 'vacuum autoclaves', and therefore have a vacuum stage. They are suitable for pre-packed items, which remain sterile when removed from the autoclave.

Type S

These are used for specific loads and instruments, and must be used strictly according to manufacturer's instructions (HTM 01–05 Decontamination in Dental Practice, Department of Health).

Industrial sterilization

This type of sterilization uses gamma irradiation (cobalt 60) to sterilize items. Items are exposed to radiation (similar to x-rays) which can penetrate the lumen of a needle. This method requires the use of very expensive/complex equipment and highly trained operators so is not carried out in the dental surgery. Single-use items such as scalpel blades, sutures, needles, etc. are sterilized by manufacturers using this method.

Disinfection

There are some items in the clinical environment, such as work surfaces, that cannot be sterilized, therefore disinfection must be used. Disinfection kills and prevents the growth of bacteria and fungi, but is not effective or unreliable against some viruses and spores.

Many different disinfectant products are available for use in the dental environment and the manufacturers' instructions should be followed with regard to their preparation, handling, and use. To ensure the disinfectant is effective for its desired use, it should be prepared to the correct strength, used in the prescribed manner, and not used beyond its shelf life.

A popular choice of disinfectant is sodium hypochlorite (bleach) and is effective against spores, hepatitis B virus, and HIV. It can be used for the disinfection of work surfaces, impressions, denture work, and in the disinfection of root canals. However, it can corrode metal and bleach clothing.

Works surfaces should be disinfected before and after all clinical procedures. Full PPE should be worn and all surfaces/equipment wiped over with the disinfectant of choice, using a disposable napkin/towel.

Impressions should be disinfected once removed from the patient's mouth and before sending to the dental laboratory. The method used will depend on the disinfectant being used and manufacturers' instructions should be followed. The following method should be adopted when disinfecting impressions:
- Once removed from the patient's mouth all impressions should be rinsed under running water to remove saliva, blood, and debris.
- The impression should then be submerged in the disinfecting solution for 10 minutes (set timer).
- Once the 10 minutes has lapsed, remove the impression and rinse once again under running water.
- The impression is then placed into a bag (if alginate wrapped in damp gauze) and attached to the laboratory card.

Medical emergencies and first aid

Principles of first aid

According to the Resuscitation Council (UK) 'medical emergencies are rare in general dental practice'.[1] Research by Girdler[2] found that even the most frequently occurring emergencies, such as faints, occur 'at rates of about 0.7 cases per dentist per year'.

Yet the GDC Standards Guidance[3] states that 'All members of staff who might be involved in dealing with a medical emergency are trained and prepared to deal with such an emergency at any time, and practise together regularly' because 'medical emergencies can happen at any time'.

Preventing a medical emergency

Whilst there is no guaranteed method to prevent medical emergencies their incidence can be limited if the dentist ensures that:
- Medical histories are taken for all patients and updated at each visit.
- For patients with complex conditions it may be necessary to liaise with their doctor in managing their dental treatment.

However, it is not just those with recognized pre-existing illnesses who may have a medical emergency. Anyone including a member of the dental team can become a casualty. It is ∴ essential that all members of the team can manage in a prompt, effective manner medical emergencies that occur within their clinical environment.

What is first aid?

- The initial care given to a casualty until the arrival of ambulance personnel, nurse, or doctor.
- Responsibility for the casualty ends when they are handed over to medical personnel.

Aims of first aid

When assisting a casualty the aims are to:
- Preserve life.
- Prevent condition worsening.
- Promote recovery.

Medical emergency guidelines

Approach and assess the casualty using:
- Danger: *do not rush in*—you risk becoming a 2nd casualty.
- Response: do they speak, groan, or flinch?
  - If they are unresponsive shout for help.
- Airway: open airway by using a chin lift.
- Breathing: hold chin lift, look, listen and feel for breath for 10 seconds.
- Casualty: if the casualty is not breathing or not breathing normally call an ambulance and commence cardiopulmonary resuscitation (CPR) (30 compressions to 2 breaths).

Principles of casualty management

- Be prepared for a medical emergency and know your role if one should occur.
- Remain calm—if you panic the casualty will panic.

- Assess any danger to you, the casualty, or other patients in the surgery and act appropriately:
  - Use standard precautions. Blood and saliva can potentially carry viruses, such as HIV and hepatitis B (see ☐ Cross infection and transmission, p.92).
- Identify the disease or condition the casualty is suffering from—if possible.
- Get help—as appropriate:
  - All members of the dental team should know their role in an emergency and should act together in assisting the casualty.
- Give immediate appropriate treatment:
  - Don't forget the importance of reassuring and calming the casualty and any companion with them.
  - Assess for shock and treat appropriately.
  - Only carry out treatment you are trained to do.
- If casualty is not going to hospital ensure they can get home safely.
- After the emergency:
  - Record the medical emergency in the Accident Book, patient notes, RIDDOR, as appropriate.
  - Reassure any other patients in the surgery who may have witnessed the event.
  - Clear and clean the area.
  - Re-stock any emergency drugs or equipment used.
  - Take care of yourself—you may feel shaken and upset by the emergency, especially if it was serious, and may benefit from talking to others or taking a break for a few minutes.
  - Carry out an audit of the emergency. Staff involved in the medical emergency should meet to run through what happened and learn from the event.

Legal considerations when dealing with medical emergencies

- No one has the right to touch or treat any one who does not wish it. This is classed as assault. Permission to treat must be sought from the casualty.
- The unconscious casualty is deemed to have given their consent so that vital functions (i.e. airway, breathing, and circulation) are maintained.
- No one can be made to go to hospital—this may be refused together with examination and treatment.

[1] Resuscitation Council UK (2006). *Medical emergencies and resuscitation. Standards for clinical practice and training for dental practitioners and dental care professionals in general dental practice.* London: Resuscitation Council (UK). Available at: ℘ http://www.resus.org.uk.
[2] Girdler NM, Smith DG (1999). Prevalence of emergency events in british dental practice and emergency management skills of British dentists. *Resuscitation* **41**:159–67.
[3] General Dental Council (2006). *Principles of Dental Team Working.* London: GDC. Available at: ℘ http://www.gdc-uk.org.

Medical emergency drugs and equipment

Although there is no regulated list of emergency drugs and equipment for all dental practices, the Resuscitation Council (UK) dental practice guidelines[1] suggest that the emergency drugs and equipment listed in Tables 6.1 and 6.2 should be available within all dental surgeries for the management of the most common medical emergencies.

Whilst other drugs and equipment are available for dental practices much of it is not considered to be first-line treatment (e.g. hydrocortisone for anaphylaxis) and will be administered, where necessary, by ambulance personnel.

Responsibilities of the dental nurse
- Be familiar with the location of all medical emergency drugs and equipment within their clinical environment.
- Be able to recognize each emergency drug and piece of equipment so they can:
  - Locate it rapidly.
  - Assist effectively in the management of a medical emergency.

Automated external defibrillators (AEDs)
The Resuscitation Council (UK) recommends that AEDs are available in all dental practices.[1] Early use of AEDs significantly ↑ survival rates in cardiac arrest and is substantially more effective than manual chest compressions (CPR) alone.

Where a practice has an AED all staff who may be involved in a medical emergency should have regular training in the use of their AED.

Storage of emergency drugs and equipment
Emergency drugs should be stored together in a purposely designed storage container. Emergency drugs and equipment should be stored safely away from patients but should be easily accessible from all clinical areas.

Each practice should designate a member of staff to check the emergency drugs and equipment at least once a week to ensure:
- There are adequate stocks of emergency drugs and equipment—including checking that oxygen cylinders are not empty.
- Emergency drugs and equipment are in date.
- Emergency drugs and equipment are in a usable, safe condition—e.g. seals and packets have not been broken or equipment damaged.

Further reading
London Ambulance Service: ℘ http://www.londonambulance.nhs.uk.

---

[1] Resuscitation Council (UK) *Medical emergencies and resuscitation; standards for clinical practice and training for dental practitioners and dental care professionals in general dental practice*. London: Resuscitation Council (UK). Available at: ℘ http://www.resus.org.uk/pages/public.htm#gen.

Table 6.1 Drugs found in an emergency medical kit

Drug	Dose	Presentation	Indication
Adrenaline (epinephrine)	1:1000, 1mg/mL 0.5Ml: adult dose 0.3mL: 6–12 years old 0.15mL: 0–6 years old	IM injection Presentation: single-dose autoinjector (EpiPen® or Anapen®) or vial with syringe	Anaphylaxis
Aspirin	300mg	Dispersible tablets to be chewed	Heart attack
Glucagon	1mg: adult dose 0.5mg: <8 years old	IM injection	Diabetic hypoglycemic coma
Oral glucose solution	N/A	Tablets/gel/powder	Low blood sugar in conscious patient
GTN	400microgram/dose given	Sublingual spray	Angina attack
Midazolam (IV or rectal diazapam may also be used)	5mg/mL 10mg/mL	Buccal Intranasal	Prolonged epileptic seizures
Oxygen	10L/minute	Black cylinder with white collar	Most medical emergencies
Salbutamol	100microgram/actuation	Aerosol inhaler	Asthma attacks

► Emergency drugs should only be administered by adequately trained and qualified personnel.

Table 6.2 Minimum equipment recommendations

Item	Description
Portable oxygen cylinder	D size with pressure valve and flow meter
Oxygen face mask with tubing	
Basic set of oropharyngeal airways	Sizes 1, 2, 3, and 4
Pocket mask with oxygen port	
Self-inflating bag and mask apparatus with oxygen reservoir and tubing	1L bag; used if staff have been appropriately trained
Variety of adult and child face masks	For attaching to self-inflating bag
Portable suction with appropriate suction catheters and tubing	E.g. the Yankauer sucker
Single-use sterile syringes and needles	
Spacer device	For use with inhaled bronchodilators, e.g. salbutamol inhaler
Automated blood glucose measurement device	
Automated external defibrillator	

▶ Emergency medical equipment should only be administered by adequately trained and qualified personnel.

The unconscious casualty

Definition
The unconscious casualty will be breathing but unresponsive to attempts to rouse them.

Causes
The main causes of unconsciousness can be memorized using the acronym 'FISH SHAPED':
- **F**ainting.
- **I**nfection.
- **S**hock.
- **H**ead injury.
- **S**troke.
- **H**eart attack.
- **A**irway hypoxia.
- **P**oisoning.
- **E**pileptic seizure.
- **D**iabetic coma.

Signs of unconsciousness
Approach casualty using:
- Danger: *do not rush in*—you risk becoming a 2nd casualty.
- Response: they will not be roused using either vocal or painful stimuli:
  - Shout for help.
- Airway: use a chin lift to open airway to allow the casualty to breath.
- Breathing: hold chin lift and check for up to 10 seconds—they will be breathing.

Aims of treatment
If an unconscious casualty is laying on their back their tongue will drop back and block their airway. This will prevent them breathing. Treatment aims to put the casualty in a safe position which:
- Allows them to breath normally.
- Allows vomit or other fluids to drain away from the mouth and prevent them choking.

Treatment
- Place the unconscious casualty in the recovery position (Fig. 6.1).
- Call an ambulance.
- Check casualty for signs of injury and deal with these as necessary (e.g. bleeding).
- Cover casualty in a blanket to keep them warm.
- Monitor casualty's vital signs continuously and be prepared to act if condition deteriorates:
  - Monitor vital signs and note your findings (Table 6.3).
  - If breathing stops, place casualty flat on their back and carry out CPR (30 compressions to 2 breaths).
- When ambulance crew arrives list your actions and patient condition to them.

Table 6.3 Vital signs that can be monitored in an unconscious casualty

Vital signs	Average normal ranges
Breathing:	
• Adult	12–20 breaths per minute
• Child	20–30 breaths per minute
Pulse:	
• Adult	60–80 beats per minute (resting rate)
• Child	60–120 beats per minute (resting rate)
Body temperature:	
• Adult	37°C (98.6° F)
• Child	37°C (98.6° F)

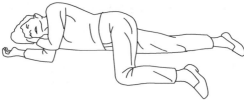

Fig. 6.1 Recovery position. Reproduced with permission from Randle J et al. (2009). *Oxford Handbook of Clinical Skills in Adult Nursing.* Oxford: OUP.

Cardiac arrest

Definition

In cardiac arrest the heart stops pumping blood around the body which ∴ starves the brain of oxygen. Within 3 minutes irreversible brain damage starts to occur.

Causes

Cardiac arrest usually occurs because of a life-threatening abnormal heart rhythm called ventricular fibrillation. Myocardial infarction (heart attack) is the most common cause of cardiac arrest occurring in this manner.

Other causes include: electrocution, drowning, choking, and trauma. There are also cases with no known cause.

Signs

Approach casualty using:
- Danger: do not risk becoming a 2nd casualty.
- Response: they will not be roused using either vocal or painful stimuli:
  • Shout for help.
- Airway: use a chin lift to open airway to allow the casualty to breath.
- Breathing: hold chin lift and check for 10 seconds—they will be not breathing or not breathing normally (agonal gasps).
  • *Agonal gasps*: casualty may make a gasping, gurgling, or snorting noise—this is not normal breathing.
- Skin may be grey.

Treatment aims

Early defibrillation increases survival rates dramatically. Most casualties will not recover with CPR alone. However, prompt CPR maintains the flow of oxygenated blood around the body until defibrillation can be commenced. For every minute without commencement of CPR or defibrillation the chances of survival are reduced by 7–10%. It is important that only trained staff use the defibrillator.

Treatment

- Call an ambulance (999 or 112 on a mobile phone in the UK).
- Commence CPR at a ratio of 30 compressions to 2 breaths (see Fig. 6.2):
  • If no pocket mask is available for rescue breaths and you are worried about infection risks then compressions alone are acceptable.
- Once CPR has commenced continue until:
  • The casualty recovers.
  • Ambulance personnel take over from you.
  • You are too exhausted to continue.

2-person CPR

If 2 people are available to carry out CPR then change over every 2 minutes (roughly 6–7 rounds of CPR) to prevent exhaustion.

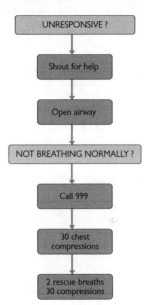

Fig. 6.2 Summary of adult basic life support. Reproduced with permission from the Resuscitation Council (UK) (http://www.resus.org.uk).

Shock

Definition
Medical shock (circulatory shock) is a life-threatening condition that occurs when the circulatory system fails and blood pressure drops to a dangerously low level. A casualty with circulatory shock may suffer from permanent organ damage or even death.

Causes
The most common cause of shock is blood loss (Hypovolaemic shock). In an adult the loss of 2 pints (1.2L) of blood can induce shock. Fluid loss from vomiting, diarrhoea, and severe burns can also result in shock.

Other causes include heart attack, severe infection, low blood sugar, hypothermia, anaphylaxis, drug overdose, or spinal cord injury.

Signs
- Pale, clammy, cold skin.
- Rapid, weak pulse.
- Shallow but rapid breathing.
- Drop in blood pressure.
- Vomiting.
- Confused behaviour.

Later signs of shock:
  - Grey-blue skin and lips (cyanosis).
  - Profuse sweating.
  - Air hunger.
  - Unconsciousness.

Symptoms
- Anxious.
- Weak.
- Dizzy.
- Thirsty.
- Nauseous.

Treatment aims
To preserve life by early recognition and treatment of shock condition.

Treatment
- Call an ambulance.
- Place casualty in supine position (flat on their back), with their feet raised if their injuries permit.
- Loosen any tight clothing, such as collars and ties.
- Cover with blanket or coat to retain body heat but do not overheat.
- Moisten lips if thirsty.
- Reassure.
- Monitor vital signs and be ready to commence CPR if needed.
- *Do not allow casualty to:*
  - Eat, smoke, or drink anything.

Anaphylaxis

Definition

Anaphylaxis is a severe life-threatening allergic reaction. It causes about 10 deaths a year in the UK. If not treated promptly it can lead to cardiac arrest.

Causes

The body's immune system decides a harmless substance is dangerous and reacts by releasing large amounts of the antibody immunoglobulin E. This triggers the release of excessive amounts of histamine which causes rapidly developing, life-threatening airway, breathing, and circulatory problems.

Common dental causes include local anaesthetic. latex, penicillin, aspirin, non-steroidal anti-inflammatory drugs (NSAIDs), and antibiotics, Non-dental causes include stings and nuts.

Signs

Signs and symptoms may vary but can include:
- Skin rash.
- Swelling (oedema) of face and airway.
- Breathing difficulties—bronchospasm, stridor, wheezing.
- Sweaty, clammy, pale skin which is cool to touch.
- Fast heart rate (tachycardia):
  - A late sign of anaphylaxis is a very slow heart rate (brachycardia).
- Low blood pressure caused by vasodilation (widening of blood vessels).
- Vomiting and diarrhoea.
- Loss of consciousness.

Symptoms

- Itching or tingling sensation.
- Dizziness and nausea.
- Breathing difficulties.
- Abdominal pain.

Treatment aims

To stabilize the patient's condition and prevent them deteriorating whilst awaiting the arrival of an ambulance.

Treatment

- Call an ambulance.
- Remove trigger if possible.
- Keep at total rest and loosen tight clothing.
- Place in a position that is comfortable for the casualty:
  - If breathing is a problem they may prefer to sit up slightly.
  - If blood pressure is very low, lay them flat and raise the legs.
- Adrenaline 1:1000 administered by casualty if they have their own EpiPen® or by dentist through IM injection (also see Boxes 6.1 and 6.2).
- Give high-flow oxygen by mask (10L/minute).
- Consider salbutamol inhaler if symptoms are mainly respiratory.
- Monitor the patient's blood pressure, pulse, and breathing.
- Be ready to do CPR.

Box 6.1 Adrenaline in anaphylaxis

In anaphylaxis the most effective first-line drug is *adrenaline*.

Adrenaline causes:
- *Vasoconstriction* which ↑ perfusion to the heart and the brain by ↑ blood pressure and reducing oedema.
- *Bronchodilation* which reverses breathing difficulties associated with anaphylaxis.
- Suppression of histamine release.

Adrenaline 1:1000 will be presented as either an autoinjector (EpiPen® or Anapen®) or a vial which will need drawing up into a syringe and should be administered by the dentist in the following doses:

Vial or Anapen® autoinjector:
- Adult 0.5mL IM.
- Child 6–12 years: 0.3mL IM.
- Child <6 years: 0.15mL IM.

EpiPen® autoinjectors are not available in 0.5mL doses and so adults should be given:
- EpiPen® (IM): 300microgram.

The dose can be repeated after 5 minutes if required.

Box 6.2 Use of autoinjectors by members of the dental team other than the dentist

Section 58 of The Medicines Act 1968 restricts the use of injectable pre-scription medicines to health professionals, such as the dentist. However this Act was modified by the *Prescription Only Medicines (Human Use) Order 1997* which created various exemptions for the purpose of saving life in an emergency.

Thus if a patient with a recognized anaphylactic condition has been pre-scribed an autoinjector, other members of the dental team can assist them administer this for the 'purpose of saving life'. However, they need to have been *suitably trained in the use of an autoinjector and be able to correctly identify that the casualty is suffering from anaphylaxis* (see also comment from HSE at: ℘ http://www.hse.gov.uk/firstaid/faqs.htm).

▶*Remember:* except for very specific situations, emergency drugs should only be administered by the dentist.

Angina

Definition

Angina is usually a symptom of coronary artery disease. Over time arterial plaque can build up on the walls of the coronary arteries. This causes narrowing of the arteries (atherosclerosis) and results in less blood and oxygen being supplied to the heart. At rest, this reduced supply is adequate to allow normal heart function without pain.

Causes

An angina attack occurs when there is a demand on the heart to work harder. This requires extra blood which the narrowed arteries are unable to supply and an angina attack occurs. Angina attack triggers include:

- Exercise.
- Stress.
- Cold weather.

Signs

- Complaint of pain or tightness in chest, left arm, jaw, or back.
- Clutching at chest.
- Belching.
- Restlessness.
- Regular fast pulse.

Symptoms

- Pain/discomfort in chest.
- Pain can radiate to the left arm, neck, jaw, and back.

Some people may also have:

- Breathlessness.
- Nausea and dizziness.
- Fatigue.

Treatment aims

To allow casualty to rest and to take medication to relieve angina pain.

Treatment

- Stop treatment:
  - Patient's medical history should record angina.
  - If not recorded, ask casualty 'Has this happened before?' and 'Have you had any medication for it?' If not a diagnosed condition treat as for myocardial infarction (see Myocardial infarction (heart attack), p.138).
- Reassure and calm.
- Sit them leaning back with knees bent (the 'W' position).
- Patient or dentist administer 1–2 sprays of GTN 400microgram sublingually.
- Pain should ease within a few minutes.
  - If casualty still has pain after 5 minutes a 2nd dose can be given.
- If the pain does not ease after 2nd dose, treat as for myocardial infarction (see Myocardial infarction (heart attack), p.138).
- Administer high-flow oxygen at 10L/minute, via face mask.

How glyceryl trinitrate works to relieve symptoms of angina attack

- GTN acts as a vasodilator (relaxes and widens the blood vessels).
- This improves blood flow to the heart muscle and relieves the symptoms of an angina attack.

Side effects of GTN can include:
- Headache.
- Dizziness.

Asthma

Definition

Asthma is a chronic condition in which the bronchi (airways) in the lungs are more sensitive than normal to becoming irritated by certain triggers. Irritation of the bronchi can cause an asthma attack. Although most people control their asthma well, asthma can be life threatening. In the UK, 1300 people a year die from asthma.

Causes

• The bronchi can become inflamed, swollen, and constricted when irritated by certain triggers. Excess mucus is also produced.
• Triggers include house dust mites, animal fur, pollen, tobacco smoke, cold air, anxiety, exercise, and chest infections.

Signs

• A wheeze might be heard, particularly on breathing out.
• Breathless with difficulty speaking or completing sentences in 1 breath.
• Coughing.
• Distress.
• ↑ respiration rate.
• Poor skin colour.

Symptoms

• Difficulty in breathing.
• Shortness of breath.
• Tightness in the chest.

Treatment aims

To reassure casualty and enable them to use an inhaler to relieve symptoms of asthma attack.

Treatment

• Calm and reassure.
• Sit the patient leaning forward—if possible rest their arms on a firm surface.
• Ventilate room and fan the casualty.
• If casualty has a salbutamol inhaler encourage them to use it or use the salbutamol inhaler in the emergency drug kit.
• If a casualty is using their inhaler ineffectively, a large-volume spacer device might be helpful.
• Encourage slow, deep breathing.
• A mild asthma attack should settle over 3 minutes. If it does not, ask the patient to use their inhaler again.

▶ Call an ambulance if:
• If this is their 1st asthma attack.
• Symptoms don't improve with medication.
• Casualty has any of the features of severe or life-threatening asthma (see Box 6.3).

Box 6.3 Features of asthma attacks

Severe asthma attack
- Symptoms will get worse quickly.
- Breathing and talking will be increasingly difficult.
- Lips and/or finger nails may turn blue.
- Rapid respiration rate >25 breaths/minute.
- Rapid heart rate >110bpm.
- Casualty shows signs of distress/exhaustion.
- Casualty has severe respiratory distress.

Life-threatening asthma attack
- Slow pulse rate (brachycardia) <50bpm.
- Cyanosis (grey-blue skin and lips).
- Slow respiration rate of <8 breaths/minute.
- Feeble respiratory effort or exhaustion.
- Confusion and altered conscious level.

Bleeding: cuts and grazes

Definition
Cuts are open wounds in the skin. Grazes are wounds where the top layers of skin are scraped off and are usually relatively minor.

Causes
Minor cuts and grazes are common injuries which are easily treated. More serious wounds may cause life-threatening haemorrhage and shock.

Signs
- Bleeding:
  - If blood spurts this suggests an artery has been cut.
  - If an object is embedded in the wound—do not remove.

Signs that give cause for concern
- Pale, cold, or clammy skin.
- Rapid and weak pulse.
- Rapid and shallow breathing.
- ↓ level of consciousness.
- Signs of hypovolaemic shock (see 🕮 Shock, p.114).

Symptoms
- Pain.
- Loss of sensation may suggest a nerve has been cut.
- Feeling faint and giddy.

Treatment aims
To assess injury and provide appropriate treatment to reduce bleeding.

Treatment
For minor cuts and grazes
- Ask casualty to apply pressure to the injury using hand or clean hand towel:
  - Bleeding will stop reasonably quickly with direct pressure.
- Wash hands and put on gloves.
- Clean wound under running water. Do not use antiseptic it can slow healing.
- Gently pat dry with dry paper hand-towel.
- Once bleeding has stopped apply a sterile dressing (e.g. a plaster, after checking that the patient is not allergic to plasters).

For severe bleeding
- Sit or lay casualty down.
- Ask casualty to apply pressure to the injury using hand or clean hand towel.
- If possible elevate the injured area above the heart to reduce bleeding:
  - If pins and needles start, lower limb to allow blood to recirculate before re-elevating injury.
- Call an ambulance.

- Wearing gloves apply pressure to the wound and firmly apply a bandage:
  - If bleeding seeps through the 1st bandage, apply a 2nd. If bleeding seeps through the 2nd bandage, remove all dressings and reapply.
- Monitor vital signs and treat signs of shock.
- If the cut has been inflicted by a used dental instrument, the sharps injury protocol should be followed.

Objects embedded in a wound

- Do not attempt to remove any objects embedded in a wound as this could cause more damage.
- To help stop bleeding do not place pressure directly over the wound but place pressure either side of the object in the wound.
- When dressing a wound with an embedded object:
  - Place dressing around the wound to stop pressure being placed on the embedded object.
  - The bandage can lightly cover the embedded object to prevent dirt getting into the wound. But make sure it is not tight over the object so that the object does not get pushed further into the wound.

Bleeding: dental haemorrhage

Definition
Dental surgery involves the cutting of tissues and a measure of bleeding is normal.

Causes
Bleeding from dental treatment is classified as:
- 1° haemorrhage—occurs at the time of dental surgery.
- Reactionary haemorrhage—occurs a few hours after dental surgery as a result of the blood clot in the wound being disturbed. Common causes of reactionary haemorrhage include:
  - Strenuous exercise.
  - Vigorous mouthwashing.
  - Drinking alcohol.
- 2° haemorrhage—occurs a few days after surgery and is caused by infection. It is a complication of a dry socket and can be very painful.

❶ Conditions such as platelet deficiency or medication such as warfarin can cause excessive bleeding and/or prevent haemostasis occurring.

Signs and symptoms
- Bleeding:
  - A small amount of blood in saliva can look like a worryingly large amount to a patient.
- Pain.

Treatment aims
To provide support to patient and allow clinician to achieve haemostasis.

Treatment
1° and reactionary haemorrhage
- Apply pressure—ask the patient to bite on a rolled-up gauze or bite pack for up to 30 minutes:
  - If patient has left the surgery and has a reactionary haemorrhage telephone advice on using a bite pack should be given and postoperative instructions re-iterated. If bleeding continues they should be advised to come back into the surgery.

If bleeding does not stop the following may be used:
- Haemostatic drug applied. Haemostatic agents can include:
  - LA adrenaline (epinephrine) applied directly to the bleeding site.
  - Absorbable haemostatic packs placed directly into the wound—e.g. oxidized cellulose (surgical) or fibrin foam.
- Sutures inserted to draw edges of surgery site together.

If these measures fail to achieve haemostasis:
- Call an ambulance.
- Monitor patient vital signs and treat for any signs of hypovolaemic shock (see 🕮 Shock, p.114).

2° haemorrhage

For a 2° haemorrhage there may also be pain. Treatment can include:

- Cleaning out the dry socket with saline or similar.
- Placing a sedative antiseptic dressing in the site, e.g. Alvogyl®.
- Prescription for antibiotics.

Burns and scalds

Definition
Burns and scalds need prompt treatment to limit the damage caused to soft tissues. (See Table 6.4 for definitions of types of burns.)

Causes
- Burns are caused by dry heat, chemicals, or irradiation.
- Scalds are caused by wet heat sources such as steam or hot water.

Signs
Superficial burns:
- Reddened skin.

Partial thickness burns:
- Reddening and blistering of the skin.
- Peeling skin.

Full thickness burns:
- Severe blistering.
- Black charred appearance.
- White appearance for chemical burns or scalds.
- Exposed fatty tissues.

Symptoms
Superficial burns:
- Pain.

Partial thickness burns:
- Pain.

Full thickness burns:
- Loss of sensation, no pain, or limited pain as nerve endings damaged.

Treatment aims
To assess severity of burn and provide treatment to minimize tissue damage.

Treatment
- Place burnt area in cool water for a minimum of 10 minutes (or until the burning sensation has stopped). Running water can be used or regularly change water as it becomes warm.
- Remove watches or jewellery near the burn if possible as swelling may occur.

Once burning sensation has stopped or if taking to hospital (see Box 6.4):
- Cover the burn to protect from it from infection. A clean plastic bag or clingfilm are good dressings as they help to retain moisture. Alternatively use a non-fluffy dressing to cover the wound.
- Monitor for signs of shock and treat as appropriate.

▶ *When treating burns do not:*
- Cover the burn with plasters or adhesive dressings, because they might cause damage to skin when they removed.
- Apply lint or fluffy dressings as they will embed in the wound.

- Apply lotions, ointments, and creams.
- Burst blisters because they function as a barrier to infection.

Box 6.4 When to send a casualty to hospital

- All full-thickness burns.
- All burns involving hands, feet, face. or genital area.
- All partial thickness burns > the size of the casualty's palm.
- All superficial burns >5x the size of the casualty's palm.
- If you are unsure of the severity of the burn.
- If the casualty is a young child.

Table 6.4 Classifying and identifying burns

Burn type	Description
Superficial	Only the outer layer of the skin is involved. Signs include redness, swelling and tenderness
Partial thickness	Several layers of skin are burnt through and blisters start to show. Burns do not blanch with pressure
Full thickness	All the layers of skin are burnt away. It may extend down through muscle and nerve endings may be damaged. Leathery, does not show any blisters. Skin affected by a full-thickness burn is numb. Will scar for life

Choking and inhaled objects

Definition
Choking occurs when breathing is suddenly impeded by something causing an airway blockage. The airway can be partly or fully blocked.

Causes
Dental patients are at particular risk of choking. They have dental instruments and materials in their mouth for extended periods of time and LA might impair the protective reflexes at the back of the mouth.

Signs
Choking
- Coughing, wheezing, or crowing noise.
- Grey coloured skin.
- Holding throat, unable to speak or cough—indicates full airway blockage.
- Cyanosis rapidly follows and the patient loses consciousness.

Inhaled object
- If object has been inhaled into the lungs, the patient might become wheezy.

Symptoms
- Difficulty breathing.
- Panic.

Treatment aims
To assist the patient to enable them to clear the object from their airway.

Treatment
Choking
- Remove obstruction if visible and safely accessible:
  - Use suction or dentist can use tweezers to grab object.
- Sit casualty upright and encourage coughing.

If no improvement:
- Encourage casualty to lean forwards and support them with 1 arm.
- Give up to 5 sharp back slaps (aim between the shoulder blades).

If no improvement and still conscious—shout for help:
- Give up to 5 abdominal thrusts—abdominal thrusts can cause internal injury. Send casualty to hospital for assessment if they are administered.

If no improvement and still conscious:
- Alternate abdominal thrusts and backslaps.

If they become unconscious:
• Call an ambulance.
• Use Danger, Response, Airway (check mouth for object), Breathing—if not breathing start CPR (30 compressions to 2 breaths) (see Fig. 6.2). If breathing, place them in the recovery position and monitor vital signs.

Inhaled object
• Reassure and calm patient.
• Arrange for patient to go to hospital for x-ray and assessment.

Diabetic hypoglycaemia

Definition
Diabetes mellitus is a condition in which the body has problems using glucose. To enter the body's cells and produce energy, glucose needs insulin. Insulin is produced by the pancreas.

Types of diabetes
- *Type 1 diabetes*—the pancreas is unable to produce any insulin and is usually treated with regular insulin injections and controlled diet.
- *Type 2 diabetes*—either the body develops insulin resistance or the pancreas doesn't produce enough insulin. Usually controlled by diet and medication.

Causes
- Hypoglycaemia is caused when blood glucose levels become abnormally low (<3.0mmol/L). Table 6.5 explains how to interpret blood glucose measurements.
- The main causes of diabetic hypoglycaemia are delayed or irregular meals, unusual exertion or exercise, stress, pain, alcohol, excessive insulin dose.

Signs
- Shaking and trembling.
- Sweating and pallor.
- Slurring of speech.
- Aggression and confusion.
- Rapid pulse.
- Normal breathing.
- Can appear drunk.

May progress to seizures, unconsciousness, and death if not treated promptly.

Symptoms
- Hunger.
- Headache.
- Poor concentration.

Diabetic people often recognize the symptoms themselves and take glucose.

Treatment aims
To ↑ the levels of blood glucose to help the patient to recover.

Treatment
- Measure blood glucose level to confirm hypoglycaemia (<3.0mmol/L):
  - Be aware: casualty may be aggressive and resist help offered.
- *Conscious patient:*
  - Give a drink of oral glucose, glucose tablets, or gel which will provide immediate glucose.
  - This can be repeated after 10 minutes if necessary.
  - When the patient is feeling better give them some carbohydrate (e.g. a biscuit) to provide longer-acting glucose.

- *Unconscious or semi-conscious patient:*
  - Call an ambulance.
  - Give buccal glucose gel or IM glucagon (see Box 6.5).
- Recheck blood glucose after administering either glucose or glucagon.

Table 6.5 How to interpret blood glucose measurements

Blood glucose measurement (mmol/L)	Meaning
2	Extremely low blood glucose
4.4–6.00	Normal blood glucose level
8.0–10.0	Normal range of blood glucose after a meal
15	A little high
20	Very high blood glucose level
33	Dangerously high

Box 6.5 Glucagon and diabetic hypoglycaemia

Glucagon ↑ blood glucose levels by:
- Liberating glucose from glycogen stores in the liver, which is then converted to glucose.
- Formation of glucose by gluconeogenesis.
- When alert and recovered give casualty oral glucose and a carbohydrate such as a biscuit.

It will be ineffective if the casualty doesn't have their own glycogen stores, e.g. anorexics or alcoholics.

Diabetic hyperglycaemia

Diabetic hyperglycaemia is a relatively uncommon cause of emergency because it generally takes a long time to develop. However, if a diabetic hyperglycaemic coma does occurs it requires prompt management.

Diabetic hyperglycaemia occurs when blood glucose levels are abnormally high and is usually caused by neglect of diet or omission of insulin therapy.

Symptoms are similar to diabetic hypoglycaemia and include:
- Headache, thirst, and blurred vision.

The signs include:
- Slow loss of consciousness.
- Dilated pupils and flushed face.
- Sluggish movements.
- Weak and soft pulse.
- Smell of acetone of alcohol on the breath (ketones).

The casualty needs an insulin injection or oral medication. If the casualty is unconscious and unable to take their own medication:
- Call an ambulance immediately.
- Keep casualty warm.

Electric shock and electrocution

Definition
Electric shock refers to the injury caused by the passage of electricity through the body. Electrocution is death caused by an electric shock.

Causes
Although lightening strikes and overhead power lines can cause electric shock the most common causes are faulty or poorly maintained indoor electrical supplies. A severe electric shock can cause cardiopulmonary arrest. The heart might restart of its own accord but prolonged respiratory arrest, resulting in hypoxia can be fatal without treatment.

Signs
- The casualty may still be in contact with source of electric shock.
- Body in spasm and unable to release source of electric shock.
- Cardiac arrest caused by ventricular fibrillation (a life-threatening abnormal heart rhythm).
- Respiratory arrest and hypoxia.
- Unconsciousness.
- Burns where the current has entered and left the body.
- Signs of severe shock.

Symptoms
In a conscious casualty symptoms might include:
- Tingling.
- Muscle spasm.
- Pain.

Treatment aims
To isolate the electricity supply and get an ambulance for casualty. To treat immediate injuries and prevent condition worsening.

Treatment
❶ Do not approach the casualty if they are still in contact with the cause of the electric shock. The electricity supply may still be live and you risk receiving an electric shock.
- Disconnect casualty from electricity. Either turn off the mains supply or push away whatever is conducting the current using an insulating material, e.g. a wooden stick—but do not put yourself at risk.
- If this is not possible ring 999 and follow their instructions.

Once the casualty has been removed from the source of electricity and an ambulance called:
- Assess the casualty using Danger, Response, Airway, Breathing:
  - If not breathing or not breathing normally commence CPR (30 compressions to 2 breaths) (see Fig. 6.2).
  - If unconscious place in recovery position, (see Fig. 6.1) monitor vital signs, treat obvious injuries such as burns, and treat signs of shock.
  - If conscious reassure, monitor vital signs, treat obvious injuries such as burns and treat signs of shock.

Epilepsy

Definition

Epilepsy is a neurological condition where there is a tendency to have recurrent seizures which start in the brain. A seizure is a brief interruption of normal electrical activity in the brain. There are a number of different forms of epilepsy and signs and symptoms may vary.

Causes

- Causes of epilepsy are varied and include genetic factors, illness (e.g. meningitis) and head injury. Epilepsy may have no known cause.
- Triggers for epileptic seizures may include: tiredness, stress, pain, alcohol, and flashing lights. It can also be caused by hypoglycaemia.

Signs and symptoms

▶ common types of epileptic seizure are detailed:

Major epilepsy (also known as tonic–clonic epilepsy)
- Patient may have an aura which is a pre-warning of a fit. They taste, smell, see, or hear something.
- Sudden loss of consciousness.
- *Tonic phase*—casualty becomes rigid, falls to the ground, may stop breathing for a few seconds, becoming blue (cyanosed).
- *Clonic phase*—casualty starts rhythmic jerking movements of the muscles. During this phase, the tongue might be bitten.
- The fitting patient might suffer incontinence and froth at the mouth.
- The casualty will stop fitting within few minutes and become limp.
- The casualty will recover consciousness but will be confused and exhausted.

Minor epilepsy (also known as absence)—more common in children than adults
- May become unconscious for a short time.
- May look blank and stare or their eyelids might flutter.
- They may continue with their pre-seizure activity, e.g. walking, but with no awareness of the dangers around them.
- These seizures can be very brief and may go unnoticed.

Treatment aims

To protect the patient from harm and facilitate recovery.

Treatment

- Stop treatment.
- Protect the patient from harm:
  - Move hazards and sharp objects, e.g. dental instruments.
  - Protect patient from harm by placing pillows or rolled blankets between them and unmovable hazards *but* do not restrain them.
- Time the length of the fit.
- Administer high-flow oxygen (10L/minute) if possible.
- After the seizure has finished place the patient in the recovery position (see Fig. 6.1).
  - They may need to sleep for some time.

- After recovery ensure casualty can get home safely, preferably with an escort.

When to call an ambulance

In general casualties who suffer an epileptic seizure will not need an ambulance. However, an ambulance should be called if:

- It is the 1st fit or no recorded medical history of epilepsy.
- Status epilepticus (seizures that last 5 minutes or longer or recur in quick succession).

Whilst awaiting an ambulance a dentist may:

- Administer IV or rectal diazepam or buccal or intranasal midazolam.
- Administer high-flow oxygen (10L/minute) if possible.
- Test blood glucose level to check not hypoglycaemic and treat for hypoglycaemia if appropriate (see 🕮 Diabetic hypoglycaemia, p.130).

Faints

Definition
Fainting (also known as syncope or vasovagal attack) is a sudden, temporary loss of consciousness.

Causes
Faints occur because there is insufficient oxygenated blood flow reaching the brain. Fainting can be caused by:
- Stress, shock, or pain.
- Fear—in very nervous patients fainting may be a result of fear about their appointment.
- Hunger.
- Prolonged exposure to heat.
- Postural hypotension (standing or sitting in one position for too long).
- Unpleasant stimuli—such as the sight of blood or dental smells.
- Hyperventilation.

Signs
- Pale skin.
- Clammy and cold to touch.
- Pulse is slow, weak, thready.
- Shivering.
- Shallow breathing.
- Low blood pressure.
- Occasionally a casualty may have:
  - Seizure-like twitching, vomiting, or incontinence.

Symptoms
- Giddy or light headed.
- Hot.
- Nauseous.
- Blurred vision or seeing in black and white.
- Altered hearing.

Treatment aims
To allow oxygenated blood to reach the brain. A patient who faints should recover quickly.

Treatment
- Place casualty in supine position (flat on their back) with their feet raised.
- Loosen any tight clothing, such as collars and ties.
- Ventilate the room.
- Monitor casualty's pulse and blood pressure.
- Administer high-flow oxygen at 10L/minute if recovery is not rapid.
- When patient starts to feel better:
  - Sit them up slowly.
  - Provide a glucose drink.
- Depending on patient's recovery, treatment may be deferred.
- Record the faint in the patient notes.

Hyperventilation

Definition

Hyperventilation means over-breathing. This involves breathing too fast and/or too deeply.

Causes

Some patients respond to anxiety and pain by hyperventilating. During hyperventilation, the respiratory rate of affected patients increases significantly, which causes the carbon dioxide (CO_2) levels in the blood to drop. This can result in spasm.

Signs

- Altered consciousness.
- Breathlessness.

Symptoms

- Anxiety.
- Weakness.
- Lightheadedness.
- Dizziness.
- Pins and needles.
- Spasm.
- Muscle pain/stiffness.
- Palpitations.
- Chest pain.
- Dry mouth.

Treatment aims

Reassure and calm casualty and assist them to breathe normally.

Treatment

- Stop all procedures immediately.
- Calmly reassure the patient and explain what is happening.
- Encourage the patient to rebreathe their own CO_2 by inhaling their exhaled breath from their cupped hands or a paper bag.
- The dentist or suitably qualified dental nurse might subsequently go through over-breathing with the casualty, explaining the symptoms as they occur to reassure them.

Myocardial infarction (heart attack)

Definition

A myocardial infarction (MI) is an interruption of the blood supply to part of the heart caused by blockage of a coronary artery. It is the number 1 cause of death in the developed world.

Causes

An MI usually occurs as a consequence of coronary artery disease. Over time arterial plaque builds up on the walls of the coronary arteries and causes narrowing. If this arterial plaque ruptures it causes a blood clot to form in a coronary artery. This starves the heart muscle of oxygen, causing it to die.

A less common cause of MI is spasm in a coronary artery which prevents the blood supply reaching part of the heart.

Signs

- Complaint of crushing pain in chest, left arm, jaw, or back.
- Clutching at chest.
- Breathlessness.
- Belching.
- Ashen skin.
- Cyanosis.
- Rapid, weak, or irregular pulse.
- Collapse.

Symptoms

- Persistent, vice-like central chest pain.
- Pain in jaw, neck, back, and down the arm—usually the left arm.
- Faintness, giddiness.
- A sense of impending doom.
- Nausea, vomiting.

Some people do not have crushing chest pain but have discomfort high in the abdomen, similar to indigestion, with neck or jaw ache.

Treatment aims

To reassure the casualty, making them comfortable and keeping them at rest whilst arranging immediate transfer to hospital.

Treatment

- Call an ambulance (999 or 112 on a mobile phone in the UK).
- Sit them leaning back with knees bent (the 'W' position).
- Offer aspirin 300mg to chew if not allergic to aspirin:
  - Can also be crushed with 2 spoons and administered sublingually.
- Give high-flow oxygen by mask (10L/minute).
- Consider analgesia in the form of a nitrous oxide (NO_2)/oxygen (O_2) mixture (Entonox®).
- Consider giving sublingual GTN spray.
- Monitor and record casualty's vital signs.
- Be prepared to carry out CPR if necessary.

The use of aspirin in MI

Aspirin is a NSAID and has a number of functions. It is a pain reliever and an anticoagulant (blood thinner).

However, in MI its function is as an antiplatelet drug. It is thought that aspirin given in an acute MI has the action of salvaging damaged heart muscle by preventing platelets clumping together and so stopping the blood clot in the coronary artery getting bigger.

Stroke (cerebrovascular accident)

Definition

A stroke (CVA) is a brain injury in which part of the brain dies through the interruption of the blood supply. When supply of blood is restricted or stopped, brain cells start to die. This can cause brain damage and possibly death. Prompt action is essential to minimize damage to the brain.

Causes

A CVA can be caused by:
- Ischaemic stroke, which is a blood clot on the brain. Blood clots usually occur because of a build-up of plaque on the artery walls which causes narrowing of the arteries. If this plaque ruptures a blood clot quickly forms.
- Haemorrhagic stroke, which is a burst blood vessel in the brain. This is usually caused by high blood pressure (hypertension) which weakens arteries in the brain.

Signs

- Slurred speech, difficulty finding or understanding words.
- Sudden loss of consciousness.
- Paralysis of one side of the face or body.
- Confusion.
- Severe headache.
- Positive FAST test (see Box 6.6).

Symptoms

- Numbness, weakness, or paralysis on 1 side of the body.
- Blurred vision.

Treatment aims

To reassure the casualty and make them comfortable whilst arranging for prompt admission to hospital.

Treatment

- Call an ambulance.
- Reassure and calm the patient.
- Place the patient into a comfortable position for them or recovery position if unconscious.
- Give high-flow oxygen by mask (10L/minute).
- Monitor and record casualty's vital signs.
- Be prepared to carry out CPR if necessary.

Box 6.6 The FAST test

The FAST test is a quick way of checking if a stroke has occurred:
- **Face:** has the casualty's face fallen on 1 side? Can they smile? Has their mouth or eye drooped?
- **Arms:** can the casualty raise both arms and keep them there?
- **Speech:** is the casualty's speech slurred?
- **Time:** if the casualty has any of theses symptoms dial 999.

Oral disease and pathology

The inflammatory process

Inflammation is part of the body's reaction to harm. This harm could be caused by a variety of things, such as bacteria and viruses (infection), trauma, or other irritants. Inflammation assists with the healing and repair of any damage caused to the body. Without this inflammatory response, wounds and infections would never heal.

Inflammation is a very complex process, which has to be well controlled by the body. If this control is lost or doesn't work properly, the body can be at risk of disease.

Inflammation is classified into 2 types—acute and chronic.

Acute inflammation
- Body's first defence against harm.
- Marked by ↑ blood flow to the injured area.
- Transfer of plasma and white blood cells causes localized swelling.
- The body's initial response triggers a complex healing process, involving the vascular and immune systems.

Chronic inflammation
- Occurs when acute inflammation is prolonged.
- Involves a wider range of cell types.
- The healing process may involve destruction of the injured tissues.

Signs and symptoms of inflammation
These can be memorized using the acronym 'SHLRP':
- **S**welling.
- **H**eat.
- **L**oss.
- **R**edness.
- **P**ain.

Periodontal diseases

Periodontology is the branch of dentistry concerned with the prevention and treatment of diseases involving the periodontal tissues. In general, periodontal diseases are infections caused by an accumulation of plaque around the gingival margin. Unlike dental caries, periodontal disease is caused by the plaque microbes that feed and multiply on *any* food debris found in the mouth.

The periodontium (peri = around, odontos = tooth) comprises the gingiva, periodontal ligament, root cementum, and alveolar bone—in addition to blood vessels, lymphatic drainage, and the nerve supply to this area (see 📖 Tooth structure, p.56).

The healthy mouth

See Fig. 7.1. The healthy gingiva (gum) is pink—sometimes with racial pigmentation—and firm. It forms a tight cuff all the way around the tooth. In between the teeth, the interdental papilla is the shape of a pyramid and, in health, extends up to the contact points of the teeth (where the teeth touch each other). The healthy gingiva often has a stippled appearance. The gingiva nearest to the crown of the tooth is not attached to the tooth or underlying bone and is known as 'the free gingiva'. Between this free gingiva and the tooth is a shallow space, known as 'the gingival crevice'. This crevice can be between 0.5mm and 3mm deep in healthy patients.

The healthy gingiva will not bleed during brushing or when the crevice is gently probed by the dentist or dental hygienist.

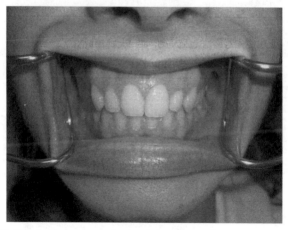

Fig. 7.1 A healthy mouth: note the triangular interdental papillae.

Plaque and calculus

Plaque

Dental plaque is a collection of micro-organisms and proteins that sticks to the teeth and other oral structures. Plaque cannot be removed simply by rinsing. Dental plaque is the major causative factor of both periodontitis and dental caries.

Formation of plaque

Plaque starts to form on the teeth almost as soon as they have been cleaned. At first, glycoproteins from the saliva stick onto the tooth and other oral surfaces. This material is known as 'the acquired pellicle' and provides a protective film for the bacteria that later on will stick to it and form plaque. During the next 7 days, if the plaque is not effectively removed, this pellicle becomes the home to predominantly round bacteria or 'cocci', mainly *Streptococcus*. As the plaque grows (as the bacteria multiply), other types of bacteria join—these might be rod-shaped *Actinomyces* or *Fusobacterium*. After 7 days, the plaque has become a very complex structure, containing many types of bacteria and proteins. Some of these proteins are made by the bacteria themselves and assist with their survival, The deeper parts of the plaque will not get any oxygen from the air that is present in the mouth so bacteria that do not require oxygen to live (anaerobic bacteria) thrive. These bacteria are of interest to period-ontologists because they are associated with periodontitis.

Plaque is usually classed as 'supragingival' or 'subgingival', as outlined in the following sections.

Supragingival plaque

Occurs above the level of the gingival (gum) margin ('supra-' = above) and is generally whitish and soft. It forms above the gingival margin, in the pits and fissures of the teeth, and around faulty restorations. The plaque is sometimes visible by eye, if there is enough of it, or it can be seen when the clinician runs a probe around the gingival margin. It is usually best seen when a disclosing agent is used—this stains the plaque various colours and is very useful when giving patients oral hygiene advice, to show them where they are missing with their brushing and flossing.

Subgingival plaque

Found within the gingival crevice ('sub-' = below), which could be as deep as 3mm, even in health. It tends to grow downwards from the supragingival plaque. Because this plaque is protected from the mouth by being in the crevice, it tends to be much more complex in nature than supragingival plaque.

Calculus

Dental calculus is a hard, mineralized substance that forms on the surfaces of teeth and other oral structures. It forms when plaque that has accumulated over a period of time and been mineralized by calcium and phosphate salts from either saliva or blood.

Although calculus does not actually cause periodontal disease, the surface of calculus is usually covered by a layer of dental plaque.

Supragingival calculus

See Fig. 7.2. This type of calculus forms above the gingival margin and is white–yellow in colour, although it can be stained darker by tobacco or foodstuffs. Because it is mineralized by salts from saliva, it is more often found near openings of the salivary glands, such as buccal surfaces of the upper molars and lingual surfaces of the lower incisors.

Subgingival calculus

See Fig. 7.3. This type of calculus forms below the gingival margin on the tooth surface. It is usually dark because often the salts that mineralize it come from the fluid within the gingival crevice and these salts are pigmented by blood products. Unlike supragingival calculus, subgingival calculus is not easily seen and usually has to be detected by the use of a probe, when it is felt as a roughness on the surface of the tooth.

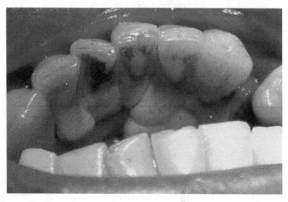

Fig. 7.2 Supragingival calculus on the lingual surfaces of the lower anterior teeth.

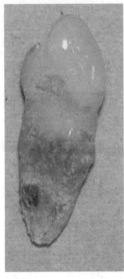

Fig. 7.3 Dark subgingival calculus on the surface of this extracted premolar.

Gingivitis

Gingivitis is inflammation of the gingivae in response to dental plaque.

Precipitating causes

If dental plaque is allowed to remain on the tooth surface and within the gingival crevice, an inflammatory reaction is triggered within the gingival tissues. This involves ↑ blood flow to the area and migration of various inflammatory cells, such as neutrophils (a type of white blood cell), from the bloodstream into the gingivae and gingival crevice. After several days, this inflammation becomes chronic in nature and different cell types migrate to the region, including lymphocytes and macrophages (more complex white cells). Chronic inflammation is limited to the gingivae and gingival crevice. If it extends beyond this region, it is classed as having progressed to periodontitis.

Recognizing gingivitis: clinical features

A patient with chronic gingivitis might notice that their gingivae bleed when they brush or floss, when they eat, or even spontaneously, such that they might notice blood on their pillow in the morning. Gingivae can become soft and spongy and the interdental papilla might become rounded and blunt (Fig. 7.4). On examination, the clinician might notice that the patients gingivae are swollen, reddened, and bleed when gently probed. This swelling, may give rise to what are known as 'false pockets' where the gingival crevice has deepened but there is no other damage.

Treatment

Providing that inflammation is still limited to the gingivae, the clinician treats gingivitis by removing any plaque-retentive factors (e.g. overhanging fillings and calculus). Educating the patient in effective cleaning techniques for the teeth and gingival margins will ↓ the chances of the condition returning.

Role of the dental nurse

- Collect the patient notes and identify the planned procedure.
- Prepare the clinical environment.
- Prepare the relevant instruments, materials, and equipment needed for the procedure, including PPE for the dental team and patient.
- If required, aspirate and retract the soft tissues to maintain a clear field of vision and remove debris.

Instruments and materials required

- Mirror, straight probe, tweezers.
- A selection of hand-held scaling instruments.
- Ultrasonic scaler and tips.
- Aspirator tip/saliva ejector.
- Cotton-wool rolls.
- Gauze.
- Contra-angle handpiece.
- Latch grip bristle brush/polishing cup.
- Prophylaxis paste.

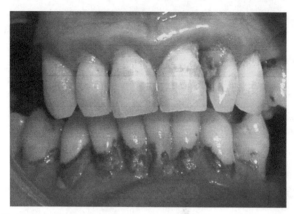

Fig. 7.4 Note the plaque accumulation at the gingival margin and swelling of the gingivae.

Periodontitis

Periodontitis literally means 'inflammation of the periodontium'.

Precipitating causes

Periodontitis occurs when the inflammatory process of chronic gingivitis is no longer limited to the gingival tissues but involves the entire periodontium. Although inflammation involving deeper tissues is not an inevitable consequence of plaque persisting in the gingival crevice, it is not known why gingivitis develops into periodontitis in some people but not in others. It might be that more virulent bacteria become involved in the crevice or that the individual's inflammatory response cannot handle the existing inflammation (as a result of an impaired immune response, psychological stress, or smoking, for example) so it spreads. Some patients have long-established gingivitis that has never developed into periodontitis.

Periodontitis is different from gingivitis in that the supporting structures of the tooth (e.g. the periodontal ligament and alveolar bone) are destroyed.

The bacteria deep within the plaque tend to be more virulent and, as the plaque grows unchecked, the number of these bacteria ↑. Some of these bacteria produce chemicals that either directly cause damage to the supporting structure of the tooth, or cause the body's (host's) own cells to cause this damage. The host cells that are present in the inflamed region, although being chiefly protective in nature, can also produce chemicals that destroy the periodontal tissues.

Recognizing periodontitis: clinical features

As inflammation persists, the collagen fibres of the periodontal ligament are destroyed and there is a migration of the epithelial attachment (junctional epithelium) along (down) the surface of the tooth—this will now be on the root surface. Migration will have formed a pocket, because what was the base of the gingival crevice has now 'moved' down the root. As this occurs, the alveolar bone supporting the tooth is also destroyed, whether by direct or indirect action of the plaque bacteria or host response, respectively, so that, when this condition is established, the patient notices loose teeth and, possibly, recession of the gingivae, as more tissue is lost (Fig. 7.5). The patient might also notice that, because of the loss of alveolar bone, their teeth have moved position (migrated).

The clinician would note a change in the contour of the gingivae, such as blunting of the interdental papillae, a more purple appearance of the gingivae, bleeding on gentle probing of the crevice, mobility of the affected teeth, and, chiefly, the presence of periodontal pockets. If a healthy gingival crevice could be up to 3mm in depth, so a depth of 4mm or more on gentle probing could indicate some periodontal destruction and the formation of 'true pockets' (or attachment loss). Radiographs would also reveal the loss of bone.

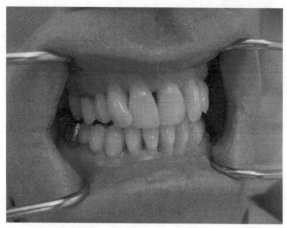

Fig. 7.5 A patient who has had severe periodontitis: there is a loss of the interdental papillae and gingival recession and some teeth have migrated.

Acute periodontal conditions

By contrast to gingivitis and periodontitis, which are chronic inflammatory conditions, patients might present with acute conditions involving the periodontium, although these are relatively rare.

Acute periodontal abscess

Precipitating causes

Might occur as an acute inflammatory reaction within an existing periodontal pocket or the gingival crevice as follows:

- An acute exacerbation (worsening) of the chronic condition, where particularly virulent bacteria might have colonized the pocket or there is a problem with the host's immune or inflammatory response.
- A result of trauma to the pocket, such as a piece of food or toothbrush bristle becoming trapped.

Recognizing an acute periodontal abscess: clinical features

This will result in the tooth becoming very tender, the gingivae becoming red, and, possibly, pus exuding from the pocket.

Treatment

Treatment might involve an incision to drain any pus that has accumulated, irrigation with chlorhexidine, and scaling of the affected root surface.

Warm salt water mouthwashes might also be advised and, if there is swelling of lymph nodes, antibiotics (usually metronidazole) might be prescribed. Antibiotics are effective against the anaerobic bacteria that often cause these problems.

Acute ulcerative gingivitis (AUG)

Precipitating causes

Poor oral hygiene, stress, smoking, and poor nutrition are often associated with this condition; it was known as 'trench mouth' in the trenches of the First World War. It was thought at that time that AUG was a contagious (catching) disease, although later studies have shown that it is not and the reason that such large numbers of soldiers suffered from the disease in 1914–18 was because of the presence of the factors listed earlier in this topic. AUG was thought to be caused by specific bacteria that invaded periodontal tissues, although now people are beginning to think it is caused by a virus because the condition is similar in nature to other viral diseases. Interestingly, despite the large numbers of virulent bacteria involved in chronic periodontitis, there is little evidence to suggest that these bacteria actually leave the pocket and invade the tissues.

Recognizing AUG: clinical features

A relatively uncommon condition, occurring mainly in young adults in the West, although a very aggressive variant is found in young children in Africa.

Ulcers occur first at the interdental papillae, which are greyish and covered with a 'pseudomembranous slough' (a layer of dead gingival cells that can be scraped off). The condition can spread to the buccal and lingual gingival margins. It is extremely painful and often accompanied by marked halitosis (bad breath).

Treatment

The treatment of AUG involves the elimination of risk factors and gentle cleaning of the affected area. If this is too painful or there is involvement of the lymph nodes, antibiotics (e.g. metronidazole) can be prescribed.

Because anaerobic bacteria were suspected to be present, oxygenating mouthwashes (e.g. hydrogen peroxide) were used in the past; these mouthwashes release oxygen and kill the bacteria.

Because of the ulceration, patients are often left with blunt interdental papillae, even following successful treatment.

Incomplete treatment or compliance can result in the condition progressing to the periodontium and becoming necrotizing periodontitis.

Diagnosing periodontal diseases

Any new patient presenting for examination and treatment must have their periodontium thoroughly examined to determine whether they have any periodontal condition. Many patients suffering from gingivitis or periodontitis are unaware that they have the disease and so might not present with symptoms.

Patients should always be examined in a systematic manner so that nothing is overlooked. This topic will outline the principles of examination and how each area is relevant to the patient with periodontal disease.

Principles of examination

Presenting complaint
Many patients with periodontitis or gingivitis are unaware of it, but patients giving a history of bleeding gums, loose teeth, drifted teeth, bad taste, or bad breath alert the clinician to the possibility of periodontitis.

Dental history
The patient's past dental history will give the clinician a clue regarding the patient's attitude to dental care and amount of care that they have already received. Information will also be gathered about how often they brush their teeth and whether they use interdental cleaning aids or mouthwashes. Reasons for previous tooth loss might also give clues about previous disease.

Social history
Smoking and stress are known risk factors for periodontal disease, so these areas should be discussed and recorded.

Medical history
A thorough medical history should be taken and examined by the clinician and reviewed at every appointment. Diabetes is a well-established risk factor for periodontitis and certain drugs also affect the periodontium, making the patient more susceptible to periodontal disease.

Clinical examination
This will involve a thorough extraoral and intraoral examination. An extraoral examination reveals enlarged lymph nodes that might result from infection, for example. Intraorally, calculus and other plaque-retaining features (e.g. overhanging restorations and poorly fitting crowns) should be recorded, in addition to the appearance of the gingivae, noting those features we described previously. The patient's plaque control should also be examined and a disclosing agent is often used to stain plaque so that areas in which plaque is present can be recorded. Tooth mobility and gingival recession should also be noted.

Specific examination

Basic periodontal examination (BPE)
To determine whether the patient has destructive periodontitis, with pocketing, it is necessary to probe the gingival crevices/pockets using a blunt probe. The British Society of Periodontology developed the BPE in 1986 as a method of screening all patients for periodontal diseases (see 📖 Basic periodontal examination (BPE), p.156).

Basic periodontal examination (BPE)

For this examination, the mouth is divided into 6 sections (sextants), not including the 3rd molars (Table 7.1).

Examination procedure

A special probe, with a 0.5mm ball-ended tip and a coloured band between 3.5mm and 5.5mm (Fig. 7.6), is used to gently probe the gingival crevices/periodontal pockets of all the surfaces of the teeth in each sextant. The deepest site is recorded for each sextant and given a score (Table 7.2); the presence of bleeding is also noted.

The term 'attachment loss' refers to total loss of periodontal attachment and includes both the pocket depth and the amount of gingival recession.

A 'furcation involvement' is bone loss involving the area in which the roots divide on a molar.

Radiographs are also used to supplement this examination by the clinician, to determine the extent of any bone loss.

BPE codes

The BPE code (Table 7.3) gives the clinician an indication of the treatment needs of the patient.

Table 7.1 Sextants

UR7–4	UR3–UL3	UL4–7
LR7–4	LR3–LL3	LL4–7

Table 7.2 The basic periodontal examination[1]

Probing depth	Code
No pockets >3mm; no calculus or overhanging fillings; no bleeding on probing	0
No pockets >3mm; no calculus or overhanging fillings, but bleeding on probing	1
No pockets >3mm (coloured band still visible), but calculus or other plaque-retention factors at or below the gingival margin	2
Pockets >3.5mm; the coloured band remains partly visible	3
Pockets >5.5mm; the coloured band disappears completely	4
Attachment loss >7mm or furcation involvement detected	*

Table 7.3 BPE codes

Code 0	No treatment
Code 1	Oral-hygiene education/instruction
Code 2	Oral-hygiene instruction, removal of plaque-retention factors, scaling, and root-surface debridement
Code 3	Oral-hygiene instruction, removal of plaque-retention factors, scaling, and root-surface debridement
Code 4	Complex periodontal treatment, in addition to treatment for code. Referral to a specialist might be required
Code *	As above

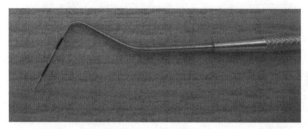

Fig. 7.6 The probe used for BPE. The first dark band is between 3.5 and 5.5mm.

[1] British Society of Periodontology (2001). *Periodontology in General Dental Practice in the United Kingdom a policy document*. Available at: ℘ http://www.bsperio.org.uk/publications/downloads/39_143748_bpe2011.pdf.

Full periodontal examination

Patients who have sextants with code 4 or * (see 📖 Basic periodontal examination (BPE), p.156) require a more thorough periodontal examination, in which each tooth in the affected sextant must be probed and the pockets and gingival recession measured at 6 points per tooth:

- Mesiobuccal.
- Midbuccal.
- Distobuccal.
- Mesiolingual/palatal.
- Midlingual/palatal.
- Distolingual/palatal.

Examination procedure

This examination is recorded on a grid known as 'a 6-point pocket chart' and the probe generally used for the examination (see Fig. 7.7) has markings at 1mm, 2mm, 3mm, 5mm, 7mm, 8mm, 9mm, and 10mm. See Chapter 10.

Classification of periodontal diseases

In 1999 the International Workshop for a Classification of Periodontal Diseases and Conditions listed the following as classes of periodontal diseases:

- Gingival diseases (G).
- Chronic periodontitis (CP).
- Aggressive periodontitis (AP)—periodontitis in younger patients (up to the age of 35 years) for which BPE scores of 4 or above would be noted, with drifting and mobility of teeth.
- Periodontitis as a manifestation of systemic diseases (PS).
- Necrotizing periodontal diseases (NP).
- Periodontal abscesses.
- Periodontitis with endodontic lesions.
- Developed and acquired deformations and conditions.

Disease is also classified according to its extent and severity:

- Localized or generalized—where in localized disease, <30% of the teeth are involved and in generalized, >30% are involved.
- Severe or moderate—depending on how much bone loss is seen on the patient's radiographs.

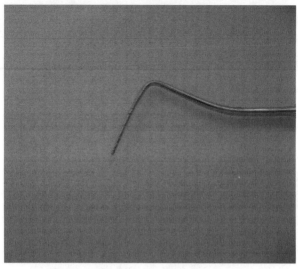

Fig. 7.7 Tip of probe used for a full periodontal examination.

Principles of treatment

Plaque

The major causative factor of the periodontal diseases is dental plaque, so treatment is geared towards removing plaque and those factors that help to retain it in the mouth (e.g. dental calculus and overhanging restorations).

Oral hygiene instruction

Treatment will usually begin with oral hygiene instruction, whereby the patient is shown how to effectively remove dental plaque at home. This will involve the use of a toothbrush and toothpaste and whatever inter-dental aids are suitable for the individual patient, such as dental floss and/ or interdental 'bottle'-type brushes.

Smoking cessation

If the patient is a smoker, smoking cessation will be discussed. Although the clinician might not be sufficiently experienced or qualified to give this type of advice, they will be able to put the patient in touch with the appropriate NHS agency or their GP to take this further, if the patient is willing to quit.

Plaque-retaining factors

Scaling

The clinician/dentist or dental hygienist then begins the important task of removing dental calculus and other local plaque-retentive factors. This is often referred to as 'scaling' and involves the removal of deposits both above (supragingival) and below (subgingival) the gingival margin. This process involves the use of sharp hand instruments, such as curettes or the ultrasonic scaler, which uses a metal tip that vibrates and effectively 'shakes' the calculus off of the tooth surface (see Figs. 7.8 and 7.9).

Root planing

For teeth that have deep pockets and deposits of subgingival calculus, these deposits are removed by a process known as 'root planing', (see Fig. 7.10) whereby not only are these deposits removed, but also some of the root cementum is removed. Very often, the cementum becomes involved in the disease process and necrotic, harbouring bacteria. Root planing is also carried out using instruments such as curettes and the ultra-sonic scaler, often under local anaesthesia.

A successful outcome of this treatment would be an improvement in the patient's oral hygiene, as demonstrated by the use of plaque indices and a resolution of inflammation, whereby swollen gingivae shrink, ↓ in bleeding on probing, and ↓ in pocket depth, which occurs as the epithelial attach-ment is re-established on the root surface.

Role of the dental nurse

- Collect the patient notes and identify the planned procedure.
- Prepare the clinical environment.
- Prepare the relevant instruments, materials, and equipment needed for the procedure, including PPE for the dental team and patient.
- Select and prepare the local anaesthetic and pass it to the dentist.
- If required, aspirate and retract the soft tissues to maintain a clear field of vision and remove debris.

Instruments and materials required

- Mirror, straight probe, tweezers.
- Local anaesthetic cartridge, syringe, and needle.
- A selection of hand-held scaling instruments.
- Ultrasonic scaler and tips.
- Aspirator tip/saliva ejector.
- Cotton-wool rolls.
- Gauze.
- Contra-angle handpiece.
- Latch grip bristle brush/polishing cup.
- Prophylaxis paste.

Raising flaps

Root planing and subgingival scaling are relatively blind procedures—that is, the clinician cannot actually see what they are doing, particularly in deep pockets. In some cases ∴ it might be necessary for the clinician or specialist periodontist to raise a flap—the gingiva is pulled away from the teeth and the root surfaces are planed under direct vision to ensure removal of all deposits. The flaps are replaced and secured with sutures (stitches).

Monitoring

Because of the chronic and progressive nature of periodontitis, it is often necessary for periodontal patients to be placed on a regular programme of scaling and monitoring.

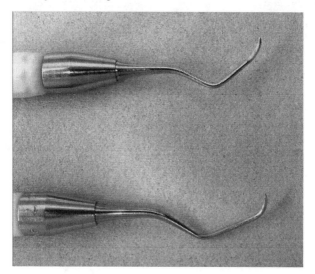

Fig. 7.8 Periodontal curettes.

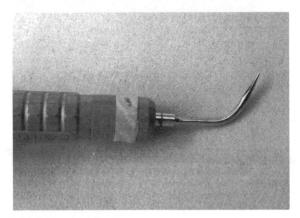

Fig. 7.9 An ultrasonic scaling tip.

(a)   (b)

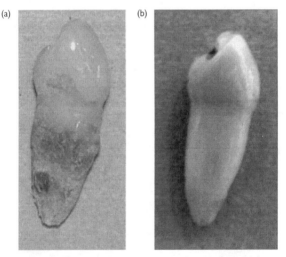

Fig. 7.10 Extracted premolar before (a) and after (b) root planing to remove subgingival calculus and necrotic cementum.

Periodontal diseases: a summary

Periodontal diseases are complex and ongoing research into how and why they occur may lead to new and more sophisticated methods of treatment. However, it is true that despite this complexity, the simple principles of treatment (as described here) are currently the most effective in tackling what is the biggest cause of tooth loss in adults in the UK.

Oral mucosal disorders

Oral mucosal lesions of interest might present as follows:
- Lumps (see 📖 Lumps in the oral cavity, p.164).
- Ulceration (see 📖 Oral ulcers, p.166).
- Inflammatory/infective disorders (see 📖 Inflammatory or infective disorders, p.168).
- White and red patches—potentially malignant (see 📖 Potentially malignant disorders, p.171).
- Pigmentation (see 📖 Pigmentation, p.171).

Lumps in the oral cavity

Overgrowths resulting from injury and trauma

These are common in the oral cavity. They are caused by irritation from sharp teeth, badly fitting prostheses, or orthodontic appliances. Common examples are outlined in the rest of this topic.

Fibroepithelial polyp

These can arise anywhere in the oral cavity but are more common on the lips, buccal mucosa, and tongue. If the polyp is found in association with gingival tissues, the overgrowth is called 'an epulis'.

Description

Most polyps are rounded, with a smooth surface. The growth is lined by normal-coloured oral mucosa and has a core of fibrous tissue. The outgrowth is usually attached to the rest of the mucosa by a broad base but sometimes by a peduncle (stalk). They are soft, but long-standing polyps are firm or rubbery because the core matures or even calcifies. Fibroepithelial polyps grow slowly and ∴ they remain small for long periods.

Removal

- Removal is undertaken for the following reasons:
  - Polyps are often bitten.
  - Aesthetic reasons.
  - Some patients request removal for pathological confirmation.
- Removal is by surgical or laser excision under local anaesthesia.
- Unlikely to recur but might leave a scar.

Denture-induced granuloma

Description

These fibrous overgrowths are found where the edge of an ill-fitting denture causes repeated trauma to soft tissue.

They are often folded several times over at the point of injury, because the denture changes position as the overgrowth ↑ in extent and size. With time, the denture becomes unstable.

Removal

- Surgical excision is indicated.
- This might result in difficulty making a well-fitting new denture.
- Tissue should be submitted for histopathological examination, to exclude any other pathological disorder.

Mucocele

Description

These are bluish lumps found mostly on the lower lip, which result from mucus retention or extravasation (leakage) from minor salivary glands into epithelium-lined sacs. The mucus that collects under the lining colours the swelling.

Injury to the mucous glands or ducts is believed to be the origin. This phenomenon leads to a cyst.

Mucoceles are more common in young people, particularly in children and young adults.

Removal
- Mucoceles might rupture, although they recur because of the presence of the fibrous sac.
- Surgical excision is indicated to eliminate mucus and the sac.
- They might recur because of trauma to the mucous ducts during surgery and healing.

Inflammatory growths

Pyogenic granuloma
Description

Pyogenic granulomas are common during pregnancy (possibly due to hormonal influence) and are also associated with poor oral hygiene. Size ranges from a few millimetres to centimetres. The surface mucosa is usually reddish-brown and might bleed if touched, at mealtimes, or during brushing. These tend to grow fairly rapidly.

Removal

Those found in pregnancy might recede but removal is indicated to enable oral hygiene procedures and repair the contour of the gum.

❶ New growths (neoplastic)

Description
- Persistent swelling.
- Present for >2–3 weeks.
- No cause found.

The most significant finding in the oral cavity is the discovery of a new growth. Early detection of such lumps might help to save a life.

Once possible causes (e.g. injury, inflammation, and infection) have been excluded, new growths should be subjected to biopsy for confirmation of whether the growth constitutes a cancer.

Clinical features include swelling, with a firm or hard base. As the growth expands, central ulceration of the lump is common.

Removal

Urgent referral is necessary and the patient should be managed by a hospital consultant following confirmation of the diagnosis.

Oral ulcers

Ulcers of the oral mucosa are common. There are many types, mostly inflammatory or resulting from immune pathology.

Traumatic ulcers

The most common type of ulcer is a traumatic ulcer, experienced by many and often caused by sharp cusps of teeth.

Treatment

Most heal in a few days and only require a covering agent to help ↓ discomfort. Removal of the cause is necessary to allow healing and the area should be kept under observation to ensure resolution. If a chronic ulcer persists for 3 weeks after removing the cause or known irritation, the ulcer should be excised and looked at under a microscope to exclude any underlying causes and malignancy.

Recurrent (apthous) ulcers

These are also common, particularly in young people. There are several varieties (minor, major, and herpetiform), classified by their size and the time taken for healing. Patients' knowledge of the history of recent recurrent ulcers might help in the diagnosis.

Treatment

Most minor aphthae last 3–5 days and don't need treatment. Major aphthous ulcers, however, last for 2–3 weeks and require medication (most commonly topical steroids) to assist healing.

Some require specialist attention. Patients are often screened to identify any underlying disorder but most patients are otherwise healthy.

In the elderly, however, recurrent oral ulceration often has a systemic cause, such as anaemia or neutropenia, or is 2° to medications. Several medications are implicated in recurrent oral ulceration.

Autoimmune causes

Other known causes of recurrent oral ulceration in the oral cavity include autoimmune disorders (pemphigus, pemphigoid, and lupus erythematosus), acquired immune deficiency (HIV disease), gastrointestinal disorders (Crohn's disease, ulcerative colitis, and coeliac disease), and haematological abnormalities (neutropenia and, rarely, leukaemia).

Neoplastic ulcers

The most significant type of oral ulcer that the dental team should be aware of is a non-healing ulcer. These ulcers persist over 2–3 weeks and do not resolve with simple remedies. They could be encountered anywhere in the mouth or in the throat.

The clinical features of a neoplastic ulcer include a firm/hard base, which results from hardening (induration) and rolled margins.

Treatment

A biopsy is mandatory and specialist opinion should be sought immediately.

The NICE guidelines (2007) require urgent referral and patients referred under the 2-week wait system are seen without delay. Confirmation of diagnosis is by biopsy.

The most common neoplastic ulcer in the oral cavity is squamous cell carcinoma.

Other investigations that must be done subsequently, include:
- Magnetic resonance imaging (MRI).
- Plain radiography of adjacent jaws.
- Computed tomography (CT) scans to assess the extent of the disease if it has spread to bone.
- A biopsy of the lymph nodes to assess any spread of the disease.
- Grading severity.

A squamous cell carcinoma is graded clinically by use of the TNM (tumour, node, metastasis) system. TNM staging helps clinicians to consider treatment options, to estimate prognosis, and compare results of treatments.

Squamous cell carcinoma treatment

Squamous cell carcinomas are treated by surgery, radiotherapy, or chemotherapy, often in combination.

Prognosis

Early or small cancers have a better prognosis than those with advanced disease. The 5-year survival rate is estimated at ~50% in most cancer centres.

Inflammatory or infective disorders

Oral lichen planus

Lichen planus is a chronic inflammatory disorder affecting the skin, oral mucous membrane, and, sometimes, genitalia.

Precipitating causes

Some people with hypertension, diabetes, or liver diseases (hepatitis) have a susceptibility to develop oral lichen planus. ♀ are more commonly affected by oral lichen planus than ♂ and the disease starts in middle age. The cause of oral lichen planus is unknown, but it is clear that there is a local immune reaction in the submucosa to an unknown antigen. Some consider it as an autoimmune disorder.

Recognizing lichen planus: clinical features

The clinical appearance of oral lichen planus is easy to diagnose if branching white lines are seen on the oral mucosa, usually bilaterally (on both sides). The areas affected in the oral cavity could involve buccal mucosa, the lateral margin of the tongue, and, sometimes, the palatal mucosa. Oral lichen planus is rare on the lips. Other varieties include desquamation of the gingivae (where the gingivae appear red and raw) and ulceration.

Treatment

Most patients are unaware that they have oral lichen planus because the mouth is asymptomatic and the disease is only found by a dentist during an examination of the mouth. Such asymptomatic patients do not require any treatment. Ulcerative lesions of lichen planus, however, can cause soreness and need long-term use of topical steroids and, occasionally, short courses of systemic steroids to obtain resolution of the eroded areas. There are other non-steroidal preparations, such as tacrolimus, which are currently being tried out for this disorder.

A diagnostic biopsy is often indicated before starting therapy and routine blood tests are performed to exclude any underlying disease that might be associated with this disorder, such as diabetes and liver disease. Ulcerative forms may be confused with discoid lupus erythematosus and a biopsy is required if such a presentation is found.

Allergy and hypersensitivity

Contact hypersensitivity to dental materials and other agents such as toothpastes and even cosmetics, could present with soreness in the oral cavity.

Recognizing allergy and hypersensitivity: clinical features

Food and drug allergies might also cause itchiness and soreness of the mucosa in a generalized pattern. It is important to differentiate allergy/hypersensitivity from conditions such as lichen planus, described earlier in this topic, that mimic it.

Investigations

Appropriate investigations include patch testing to dental materials and food allergy testing (radioallergosorbent test [RAST]).

Orofacial granulomatosis (OFG)

OFG often presents as a lip swelling. In practice, this term is imprecisely used for many disorders.

Precipitating causes

Oral granulomatous lesions resulting from tuberculosis, Crohn's disease, or sarcoidosis should be considered in the differential diagnosis and appropriately investigated. If the disease is limited to the mouth, with no evidence of systemic disease, the term 'OFG' is appropriate. Such localized granulomas are attributable to some specific microbial agents or food allergies, such as benzoate and cinnamaldehydes used as preservatives or flavourings.

Glossitis

Precipitating causes

Depapillation (smoothness) and a glazed appearance of the dorsal surface of the tongue are often encountered in the tropics and in vegetarians because of deficiencies of micronutrients, such as iron, vitamin B12, folate, and zinc.

Recognizing glossitis: clinical features

The deficiencies can be detected by a routine blood screen. Other pathological conditions that must be considered in the differential diagnosis are geographic stomatitis (erythema migrans), which demonstrates localized depapillation surrounded by a white/buff-coloured line, or sometimes oral submucous fibrosis. Erythematous candidiasis can also contribute to central depapillation of the tongue.

Treatment

Management of micronutrient deficiencies should be in consultation with the patient's physician, mostly by supplementing the deficient micronutrients, as well as supported by dietary advice.

Infections

Bacterial, fungal, and viral infections of the oral cavity occur at all ages.

These conditions often result in a sore mouth, from mucocitis and oral ulceration.

Investigations

Chronic infections, such as syphilis and tuberculosis, mostly cause chronic persistent ulcers that require biopsy and other special tests (e.g. serology for syphilis and a chest x-ray and sputum analysis for tuberculosis) to confirm the underlying diagnosis. Biopsy might show the presence of granulomas, with or without caseation (change in consistency to a soft, cheese-like form).

Fungal infection

The most common fungal infection of the oral cavity is candidiasis. Many different forms of candidiasis are seen in the oral cavity, and also at the corners of the mouth (angular cheilitis). Swabs, smears, and rinses of the mouth might help confirm colonization by *Candida* and assess sensitivity to a range of antifungal agents that are available to manage this condition.

Most people with candidiasis might have an underlying systemic disease (e.g. diabetes, anaemia, or HIV) and it is prudent to arrange appropriate blood investigations, particularly if frequent and recurrent infections are found or therapy does not eradicate the disease. Denture wearers are likely to harbour oral candidiasis and should be instructed on proper denture hygiene.

Viral infection

Viral infections of the oral cavity commonly manifest as vesiculobullous (blister-like) lesions, which later produce $2°$ ulceration. Oral infections caused by herpes simplex (HSV type 1) are commonly encountered in children and might present as inflammation of the gingivae and other parts of the mouth. Recurrent HSV infection in adults is occasionally encountered in clinical practice and affects the attached gingivae and hard palate in people with various immune deficiencies.

Recurrent herpes labialis (cold sores) in lips are found in 20–30% of people who had a $1°$ herpes infection. *Herpes zoster* (shingles) might cause an eruption restricted to the pathway of the trigeminal nerve in a unilateral fashion.

Other examples of viral infections include cytomegalovirus (causing oral ulcers), Epstein–Barr virus (causing hairy leucoplakia), and HHV8 (causing Kaposi's sarcoma, mostly in HIV-seropositive individuals).

Potentially malignant disorders

Recognizing potentially malignant disorders: clinical features

White and red patches of the oral cavity may be attributable to many causes, but some of these may have the potential to change to cancer and are known as potentially malignant disorders. Leucoplakia (white) and erythroplakia (red), mostly caused by tobacco use, carry such potential risk. Some could have a mixed appearance, referred to as 'erythroleukoplakia'. The surface of white and red plaques could be flat, nodular, or verrucous.

Investigation

To assess the risk of these disorders, a biopsy is essential to enable a microscopist to grade the lesion.

Treatment

Most moderate and severe lesions need excision by scalpel or laser.

Prognosis

Over time, cancer might develop in ~5% of potentially malignant disorders and ∴ it is essential to advise patients to do the following:
- Quit tobacco use.
- Eat fruit and vegetables.
- Arrange 6-monthly or yearly follow-up.

Pigmentation

Brown/black pigmentation (blood pigments)

Caused by the following:
- Haemorrhage following injury (including suction injury) and surgical interventions.
- Submucosal haemorrhage because of a haemorrhagic disorder—this can be indicative of a platelet disorder and should be investigated by a blood screen.

Brown pigmentation (pigmented gums)

- Most commonly observed in dark-skinned people and smokers because of melanosis.
- Localized pigmentation in the mouth could result from postinflammatory changes, deposition of amalgam particles (amalgam tattoo), or mucosal tattooing.
- Associated with some systemic disorders, such as Addison's disease—such cases would require investigation in a specialized endocrine unit.
- Oral pigmentation is also sometimes present in HIV disease.
- Some medications contribute to oral pigmentation.
- The most serious presentation is that resulting from melanoma—fortunately, these are rare in the oral cavity.

Swelling

Swellings in the salivary glands

Acute

The most common acute swelling of salivary glands in children is caused by paramyxovirus infection, resulting in mumps; it is less often encountered in adults.

Ascending bacterial infections are often found in dehydrated or debilitated patients and a purulent discharge from the salivary duct is diagnostic. Pus taken on a swab can be sent for culture and sensitivity. After a surgical procedure close to any salivary duct opening, an acute swelling might arise because of surgical misadventure and result in blockage.

Recurrent

Recurrent swellings of salivary glands are seen in 'meal-time syndrome' because of partial obstruction of the duct system by salivary calculi (stones). Most calculi can be detected by plain radiography or ultrasound.

Persistent

Common in metabolic conditions, such as diabetes and chronic alcoholism.

Persistent swellings should be investigated by imaging (ultrasound, MRI, and sialography) and biopsy with fine-needle aspiration (FNA) to exclude any neoplastic growths of salivary tissue (adenomas and adenocarcinomas) and lymphomas. Lymphomas and swellings (cystic) of salivary glands are more common in HIV disease or autoimmune diseases (Sjögren's syndrome).

Enlargement of lymph nodes

Enlargement of lymph nodes in the orofacial region commonly results from mouth and jaw infections.

A malignant tumour might spread to the regional lymph nodes and the patient should be investigated for any unknown 1° tumour by visual inspection, palpation, endoscopy, and, if indicated, imaging.

If a 1° tumour cannot be found, the swollen lymph node is investigated by ultrasound and FNA. Such investigations also help in the discovery of lymphomas. Examples of specific disorders that might affect lymph nodes in the head and neck region include tuberculosis, sarcoidosis, and several types of leukaemia.

Jaw swellings

Swellings of jaws could be inflammatory because of hamartomas, cysts, or neoplastic conditions. Osteomyelitis of jaws is caused by untreated or inadequately treated dental infections, mostly by anaerobes or in predisposed people who have had prior radiotherapy to the head and neck region. Plain radiographs are diagnostic. Hamartomas in jaws (odontomes) are encountered in young people and arise because of malformation during odontogenesis from the tooth germ.

Dental cysts are often present as localized swellings in tooth-bearing areas of jaws. They could arise because of chronic periapical infection or cystic changes during development of a tooth germ. Some cysts are incidental findings during routine radiography.

Neoplasms in jaws are mostly odontogenic in origin and benign in nature. As a result, they expand slowly. These tumours mostly appear radiolucent on plain radiographs and cone-beam CT imaging is helpful to determine the extent of bone expansion. A diagnostic biopsy is necessary to determine the type of tumour because there are many varieties of odontogenic tumours. Very rarely bone metastasis from other organs can be found in jaws, but the clinical presentation is more likely to be numbness in the face or a pathological fracture.

Dental caries

Dental caries: an overview

Dental caries is a multi-factorial disease affecting the dental hard tissues enamel, dentine, and cementum. This is a disease which affects most of the population at some stage during their life. However, nowadays, it mainly affects specific vulnerable groups such as inner-city children, persons with special needs, and the socially deprived communities.

There are also the elderly who have reduced salivary flow, for example due to medicines they have to take. A reduced salivary flow can also occur following radiotherapy. Such patients are also more susceptible to dental caries. Dental caries is a plaque-related disease in that without dental plaque, the disease cannot affect the dental hard tissues.

Over time and with the influence of the additional factors listed under 'Aetiology' the tooth tissue will begin to break down, which in turn may lead to a cavity forming within the tooth. So how does this occur?

Aetiology

The factors involved are
- Bacteria.
- Fermentable carbohydrates (sugars).
- Tooth.
- Time.

All these factors must come together to initiate caries. Absence of any 1 factor prevents caries from developing. This property can be used in prevention. These 4 factors can be illustrated diagrammatically with 4 overlapping circles (see Fig. 7.11).

Bacteria

Specific bacteria, most important of which are *Streptococcus mutans* and lactobacilli acting on fermentable carbohydrates in foods, produce acids. Whilst the *Streptococcus mutans* initiate the process, the lactoballi thrive within the acidic environment.

Fermentable carbohydrates

Some bacteria have the ability to convert sugars such as sucrose, glucose, and fructose into acid. If this acid is left on the tooth it can cause the demineralization of the enamel

Tooth

Presence of plaque is necessary for caries to occur. Therefore, any areas or conditions favouring plaque accumulation can lead to a higher risk of caries. The vulnerable sites are
- Pits.
- Fissures.
- Approximal surfaces.
- Cervical margins.
- Exposed root surfaces (in older adults).
- Medically compromised patients, especially those with a reduced salivary flow in patients undergoing radiotherapy.

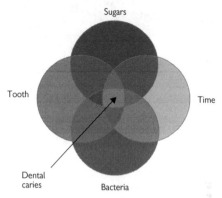

Fig. 7.11 The aetiology of dental caries.

Time

The more frequent the intake of sugars the more the tooth is exposed to an acidic environment and the natural pH level within the mouth drops. The normal level is around 7; however, the critical level where demineralization takes place is around 5.5. This can be further explained by what is known as Stephan's curve (see 🕮 Stephan's curve, p.176).

Types of caries

Depending on the tissues affected, caries can be termed enamel caries, dentine caries, and cementum caries. Based on the site of the tooth affected, caries can also be described as pit and fissure caries, smooth surface caries, and root caries.

It should not be forgotten that dental caries can also occur in children—in some cases this can be in the form of what's known as bottle caries and rampant caries.

Bottle caries

Bottle caries occur in a child's deciduous dentition, for example, in young children who fall asleep with a sweet drink in a bottle. Another way is if a child consumes several sugary drinks during the day, again from a bottle. Bottle caries can affect the teeth in general, however it does tends to affect the maxillary teeth more due to the position of the bottle.

Rampant caries

Rampant caries is more aggressive and can affect several teeth and many different surfaces. Individuals who consume a high quantity of sugar can be at risk.

Those who have undergone radiotherapy to the head and neck to treat cancer can also be at risk if the salivary glands have been affected, ∴ reducing the flow of saliva. This condition alone is known as dry mouth or medically known as xerostomia.

Stephan's curve

The normal pH level within the oral cavity is around 7. For demineralization to occur, the pH has to ↓ below 5.5. Salivary buffers can maintain pH above 5.5 thus preventing demineralization.

During initial stages, the process can be reversed as the pH returns to normal. This is remineralization which is aided by fluoride ions (see 📖 Fluoride, p.180). Therefore, caries is a dynamic process of demineralization and remineralization.

Stephan's curve (see Fig. 7.12) shows how pH drops when a sugary drink is taken. The pH has to fall below 5.5 for demineralization to occur. It takes about 45 minutes for the pH to recover. There are individual variations depending on a number of factors such as the quantity and quality of saliva.

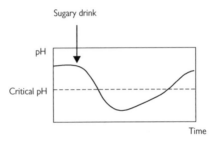

Fig. 7.12 Stephan's curve.

The process of dental caries

Initially the individual may not be aware that the caries process has started. The first sign of a new carious lesion will be a chalky white spot on the tooth. This is known as a *white spot lesion*.

This means that the *enamel* has undergone an element of demineralization. As this process continues the area may then discolour and turn brown. If left this could develop in to a cavity.

If the brown spot appears rather shiny this may suggest that the process of demineralization has stopped. This is known as arrested caries.

At this stage the patient will feel *no pain or discomfort* as the enamel does not contain any nerves or blood vessels. Once a cavity has formed the damage to the tooth will be permanent.

As the dental caries progresses the *dentine* will then be affected and ∴ becomes involved. At this stage the cavity may be more noticeable.

As the process continues the dentinal tubules become exposed. As these have a direct passage to the pulp or the nerve the patient may now experience pain and discomfort especially when eating and drinking hot or cold food or indeed sweet food.

As the dentine is softer this will undermine the enamel and possibly cause the tooth to fracture.

As the dental caries progresses further towards the *pulp* the pain may intensify. Once the pulp chamber has been reached the pulp can become infected. This can develop into a very painful condition known as *pulpitis*. At this stage the pain will be *intense*.

Again, if left the pulp will then *die*. Thus the pain will no longer be present. If the patient does not receive any treatment a dental abscess may start to form around the apex of the tooth. This is known as a *periapical abscess*.

Note: dental charting

When a clinician examines a patient and records findings, it is common practice to chart all carious lesions. The dental nurse has to be familiar with dental charting (see Chapter 10).

Diagnosis

In some cases dental caries can be diagnosed by carrying out a visual inspection in the mouth. For this to be done effectively, a clean tooth, good lighting and good eyesight are necessary. A dry surface makes it easier to identify early white spot lesions. The dental nurse may assist the dentist by passing a cotton-wool pledget on a pair of tweezers to dry the area.

Radiographic diagnosis

Not all lesions are visible to the naked eye. For example, lesions on approximal surfaces of teeth may escape detection. In addition, the extent of the lesion cannot be estimated by looking at carious teeth. Radiography is a good aid. The most useful type is a bite-wing radiograph (see Fig. 7.13 and Table 7.1).

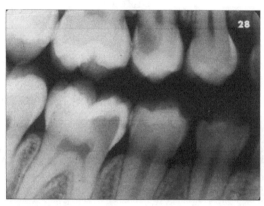

Fig. 7.13 Caries visible on a bite-wing radiograph, note the radiolucent (dark) areas associated with UR5 LR6, for example.

Fibreoptic transillumination (FOTI)
A bright light transmitted via a fibreoptic cable is shone at the approximal surfaces of the tooth. Carious lesions appear as dark shadows.

Note: Certificate in Dental Radiography

Dental nurses can get additional training in dental radiography. Many dental schools and hospitals offer courses leading to a Certificate in Dental Radiography. Certificated dental nurses can take radiographs under the direction of a dentist.

Treatment
We know that when the natural structure of a tooth is lost it will not repair itself. Therefore the aim of treatment is to preserve the remaining tooth structures and prevent further destruction of the tooth.

The easiest way to replace the missing structure would be by placing what is known as a restoration or filling. The dental caries is removed and the cavity is cleaned and shaped. Dependent on the size and location of the cavity, it can be filled with amalgam or composite.

If the dental caries has destroyed too much of the tooth then a crown may be required. Depending on the location and the amount of remaining tooth tissue these will made from gold, porcelain, or porcelain fused to metal.

Should the pulp be exposed then a root treatment may be required. This is when the nerve in the centre of the tooth is removed. The canals will be cleaned, shaped, and, at the appropriate time, filled. A crown may then be placed to support the remainder of the tooth.

As a last resort, a tooth with extensive caries may be extracted (see 📖 Surgical extractions, p.300).

Prevention

Fermentable carbohydrates in foods are necessary for initiation of caries. In addition, the frequency of dietary intake is also an important factor because the more frequently a cariogenic diet is taken, the more frequently the pH falls below the critical value of 5.5 which is needed to initiate demineralization (see 📖 Stephan's curve, p.176).

This provides an opportunity to advise patients about eating a healthy diet and avoiding excessive consumption of foods favouring plaque accumulation, i.e. cariogenic foods, including all sugary foods and starch. Sticky foods are more cariogenic.

Fluoride

Fluoride helps to prevent dental caries. Fluoride acts in several different ways: by reducing solubility of enamel by becoming incorporated into the enamel; by promoting remineralization; and by ↓ acid production by cariogenic bacteria.

Fluoride comes in many different forms. The commonest is toothpaste. Most brand name toothpastes contain an element of fluoride amongst the ingredients. It is important to remember that children's toothpaste will differ from adults and therefore the correct toothpastes should be used depending on age (Table 7.4).

An effective public health measure is to add fluoride to drinking water. However, there are those who object fluoridation of water on environmental and for reasons of personal choice.

Additional measures come in the form of fluoride drops and fluoride tablets.

Oral hygiene

A good oral hygiene routine should be adopted to help minimize the risk associated with both dental caries and, more importantly, periodontal disease. More detailed information on oral hygiene can be found on 📖 Oral hygiene instruction, p.252.

Diet

With regards to diet, the frequency of sugar is more important than the amount of sugar consumed. The more frequently teeth are exposed to an acidic environment; the more likely dental caries are to occur. Therefore, minimizing snacking is recommended. The best way to assess this is to ask the patient to complete a diet sheet or diet analysis. This can be over a period of 4 days and it is best to include a weekend as an individual's diet can change during this time (see 📖 Oral hygiene instruction, p.252).

Table 7.4 Recommended fluoride content for children in toothpaste

Age	Fluoride content
0–3 years	1000ppm (smear)
3–6 years	1350—1500ppm (pea-sized amount)
6+ years	1350—1500ppm (pea-sized amount)

ppm, parts per million.

Patient care and management

Close-support dentistry

The concept of 'team dentistry' has been around for several years and is ∴ by no means a new idea.

It is fair to say that a dentist will benefit from having a skilled dental nurse who provides fundamental chairside support to ensure smooth and efficient running of a busy day-to-day surgery.

It is essential that the dentist and dental nurse can work together as a team to achieve the following:

- Improve patient comfort and make a patient more relaxed and treatment ∴ relaxed.
- ↓ the time treatment takes by effectively passing instruments.
- ↓ stress and fatigue for the dentist with excessive body movement.
- Provide a high standard of patient care.
- ↑ the role of the trained dental nurse and promote greater job satisfaction and motivation.
- Provide effective techniques for moisture control and improve vision for the dentist nurse and ↑ comfort for the patient.
- Improve the dentist–patient relationship.

Nevertheless, the dentist must never take the dental nurse for granted or fail to appreciate the importance of their role.

Zoning

It is essential that both the dentist and dental nurse are seated in the appropriate positions in relation to the patient. Basic concepts are required for the practice of comfortable 4-handed dentistry. The 'clock' concept is one of the best ways to identify the correct position for the dental team.

Imagine a circle placed over the dental chair with the patient's face in the centre of the 'clock face' and the top of the patient's head at '12 o'clock'. The face is divided into 4 zones (Fig. 8.1).

Static zone
This zone is located behind the patient.

Dental nurse zone
This is the area allocated for the dental nurse. The instruments and materials will take up a great deal of this area, depending on the surgery design.

Transfer zone
This is the area in which dental instruments and materials are passed (over the patient's chest).

▶ Instruments should not be passed over the patient's face because this could be dangerous if instruments were to fall and might also cause a patient to start worrying, especially if passing local anaesthetic apparatus.

Operator's zone

This is the area in which the dentist will work. The dentist will move within the areas, depending on the treatment being carried out.

Although these positions are not set in stone, this model encourages good practice among the team.

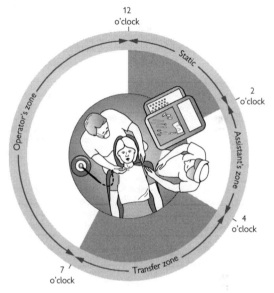

Fig. 8.1 Zoning.

Positioning the patient

Role of the dentist

The dentist should greet the patient in a manner that is appropriate to the situation. This might be with a handshake and verbal communication (e.g. 'Good morning, Mr Smith'). After the patient is seated and comfortable, it is normal for the dentist to move to the '7 o'clock' position so that face-to-face communication can take place. The dentist should never sit behind the patient during long conversations. Not only does this appear rude, but also the patient might feel uneasy about what is going on behind them.

Role of the dental nurse

Once the dental nurse has called the patient by name, they might, if necessary, assist them into the surgery. The dental nurse then takes the patient's bag and coat and places them in a safe location so as not to cause a trip hazard. If the patient is elderly and finds movement difficult, it might be necessary to assist them in moving to the dental chair and, indeed, placing their legs on the chair. ► Never assume the patient needs assistance, it is always best to ask. The older generation can be fiercely protective of their independence.

Once seated in the dental nurse chair the dental nurse will listen to the conversation between the patient and the dentist. The dental nurse will remain in position but might turn to face the dentist and patient. It is not uncommon for the patient to ask the dental nurse questions relating to the impending treatment and these should answered in a language that the patient understands. If the dental nurse is unsure, they should be addressed to the dentist.

Moisture control

One of the roles of the dental nurse during treatment is to provide effective moisture control. This is important for many reasons:

- Placing a filling (restoration) into a wet cavity will normally result in the restoration not staying within the cavity.
- When using materials that require an etched surface, such as composite, it is crucial that the area is kept dry after the etch has been removed.
- Contamination by saliva will affect the prepared surface and result in the area needing to be re-etched.

Methods of moisture control

There are many ways in which moisture can be controlled within the patient's mouth, e.g.:

- High-volume aspirator.
- Saliva ejector.
- Cotton-wool rolls.
- Cotton-wool pledgets.
- Dry guards.
- 3-1 syringe.
- Rubber dam.

High-volume aspiration

High-volume or wide-bore aspirators are the most commonly used type of aspirators in dentistry. The device is normally held in position by the dental nurse. The high-volume aspirator will remove saliva, debris, and water from the patient's mouth during restorative procedures in which an air turbine is used or ultrasonic cleaning for which water will be present in large quantities within the oral cavity. Depending on the location of the tooth, the cheek can also be retracted to aid vision. However, the dental nurse should be aware of the location of the gag reflex and try to avoid this area.

Low-volume aspiration

Low-volume aspiration includes the use of a saliva ejector. This does not have the same aspiration capabilities as the high-volume aspirator so it is normally used in conjunction with the high-volume aspiration tip. A saliva ejector can be held by the patient, especially if a rubber dam is used because the patient sometimes finds it difficult to swallow when this is in place. The patient can remove saliva from the back of their mouth without disturbing the dentist, which can be advantageous.

A flange saliva ejector can also be used, especially in a patient with an active tongue. Not only will saliva be removed, but also the tongue will be protected. Again, this device can be held by the patient or dental nurse.

Cotton-wool rolls

Cotton-wool rolls can be placed in the buccal sulcus (in between the cheek and gingiva), especially near the salivary ducts, by the dentist. These will absorb moisture but must be changed frequently.

Cotton-wool pledgets

Cotton-wool pledgets are small cotton-wool balls that can be used to dry the cavity before a lining or restoration is placed.

Dry guards

Dry guards, such as cotton-wool rolls, can be placed in the buccal sulcus, especially around the areas that the parotid salivary ducts exit into the mouth. Again, their main function is to absorb moisture from the mouth.

3–1 syringe/nozzle

A 3–1 is a multifunctional piece of equipment:

- It can be used with the air function to direct a cool flow of air into a cavity to dry.
- The water facility can be used to clean the cavity of small tooth fragments and debris.
- In some cases both facilities can be used together.
- Tips can be disposed of after each patient.

Rubber dam

If a rubber dam is applied correctly, it is an effective method of moisture control. The application of a rubber dam will have the following advantages and benefits for the dentist, dental nurse, and patient:

- Maintains a dry field.
- Retracts soft tissues.
- Prevents materials from falling into the oral cavity.
- Aids infection-control techniques by ↓ aerosol spray from the oral cavity.
- ↓ contamination to the tooth.
- Provides a visual contrast—between the tooth and the rubber dam.
- Provides patient management.
- ↑ patient comfort.
- ↑ safety of removal of amalgam fillings, as it prevents the patient from swallowing even small amounts of filling material
- ↑ the success of restorations—by providing all advantages of this list.

Angina

The term 'angina' is used to describe pain in the chest that is caused by an insufficient blood supply to the heart muscle, i.e. when the blood supply to the heart is insufficient to meet the oxygen demands of the heart muscles. The usual cause of angina is narrowing of the arteries by fatty products deposited around the walls of the blood vessels (atherosclerosis). The annual mortality rate for angina is ~4%.

↑ risk

The following are risk factors for angina:
- Smoking.
- Diabetes mellitus.
- ↑ blood cholesterol.
- A family history of ischaemic heart disease (IHD).

Precipitating causes

Angina typically occurs if extra demands are placed on the heart, e.g.:
- Physical exertion, such as climbing stairs.
- Emotional stress, anxiety, and anger.

Signs and symptoms

Pain from angina can be very frightening for the patient, e.g.:
- The chest feels constricted, tight, and heavy—it feels difficult to breath and pain typically comes from behind the breast bone (sternum).
- In severe cases, the pain can typically radiate to the left arm and sometimes to the mandible or teeth.

Stable angina

Occurs only on exertion and is relieved by rest, within 10 minutes, making the condition reversible. Also, there will have been no changes in the frequency or duration of the symptoms within the previous 60 days.

Unstable angina

The symptoms occur randomly and have sudden onset.

Dental implications

- Good pain control, by use of a local anaesthetic, is needed.
- The patient should have minimal anxiety.
- Appointments should be short.
- Patients already using glyceryl trinitrate (GTN) could be given one spray prophylactically (as prevention).
- Oxygen should be readily available.
- If symptoms arise during treatment, the procedure should be stopped and GTN administered immediately, in addition to 100% oxygen.
- If symptoms persist, the emergency services should be called.

Asthma

See also: 📖 Asthma, p.120.

Background
- Asthma affects 5.2 million people in the UK.
- 1.1 million children are receiving medical treatment for asthma.

Definition
Asthma is a common, under-recognized chest condition, which involves reversible narrowing of the airways, resulting in wheeze or coughing and difficulty in breathing. The linings of the walls swell and become inflamed. Sometimes a sticky mucus or phlegm makes the tubes even narrower.

Patients with severe asthma might tend to make light of the severity of their condition. It is important to remember that this is a life-threatening condition and must be taken seriously.

Risk factors
Attacks are commonly triggered by the following:
- Stress, emotion, and anxiety.
- Exercise.
- A 'cold' or chest infection.
- Allergic responses.
- Exercise.

Asthmatic patients often have early morning dips in the efficiency of their breathing.

Signs and symptoms
- Wheezing when breathing—sounds louder when breathing out compared with breathing in.
- Tightness of the chest.
- Breathlessness and difficulty getting air into the lungs.
- The patient sits or stands with their hands on their thighs to help the muscles used for breathing.

Medicines and devices used for asthma
- Inhalers.
- Steroids.
- Spacers and nebulizers.

Dental implications
Symptoms can develop during a course of treatment because of the following:
- Pain.
- Anxiety.
- Stress of a long procedure.
- Allergens or air pollutants in the surgery.

Epilepsy

See also: 📖 Epilepsy, p.134.

Background

- ~0.5 million people in the UK have epilepsy.
- 52% of people with epilepsy are seizure-free because of medication.
- Some become free of the condition as they get older.

Definition

Epilepsy can affect anyone. It describes a condition in which there are abnormal, intermittent periods of electrical activity in an area of the brain, which results in seizures. There are different types of epilepsy, depending on the part of the brain affected.

Legal requirements

In some cultures epilepsy still carries a stigma. Epilepsy is covered by the Disability Discrimination Act.

Precipitating causes

Epilepsy can be caused by the following:
- Head injury.
- Lack of oxygen to the brain, e.g. during a faint.
- Tumour.
- Metabolic cause, such as hypoglycaemia and hyperglycaemia.
- Infections, such as encephalitis and HIV.
- It might be idiopathic (for no known clinical reason).

Seizures

- The patient might experience a brief warning or 'aura', which might involve their sight, hearing, or smell and alerts them to the oncoming fit. It might be a strange feeling in the stomach, a sensation, or experience (e.g. deja vu).
- The seizure might have different signs, as follows:
  - Absence—a brief pause, with sudden onset and termination.
  - Tonic–clonic—sudden onset, loss of consciousness, limbs stiffen, and then jerk.
  - Myoclonic—a sudden muscle spasm throwing the person to the ground.
  - Atonic—a loss of muscle tone, so the person becomes floppy and flaccid.

Most people can control the symptoms of epilepsy by use of prescribed medicines.

Dental implications

Dental staff must be aware that a patient has epilepsy. Seizures can be initiated by the following:
- Pain.
- Anxiety.
- Flashing lights.

Diabetes

See also: □ Diabetic hypoglycaemia, p.130.

Risk factors
- Obesity.
- High blood pressure.
- Age.
- Family history.
- Ethnicity.

Causes

Diabetes mellitus affects the control of the glucose level in the blood. There are 2 main types (see Table 8.1). Both types result in ↑ glucose levels in the blood and are treated by medication to control the glucose level. Insulin is administered—this is a hormone that helps the cells of the body to take up excess glucose.

Signs and symptoms in untreated patient
- ↑ thirst.
- ↑ need to urinate.
- Extreme tiredness.
- Weight loss.
- Eye damage.
- Slow wound healing.

Early detection and treatment quickly relieves symptoms and also ↓ the chances of developing serious health problems.

Dental implications
- If an insulin-dependent diabetic patient misses a meal (having taken the glucose-lowering medication), they will experience ↓ blood glucose. This can become critically low, causing a hypoglycaemic episode.
- Early recognition and treatment is crucial, because these events can be (and frequently are) fatal.

Precautions
- Treat patients at the most suitable time, after a meal and medication.
- Treat with the least amount of trauma, to improve healing.
- Have glucose ready for a hypoglycaemic event.
- Be aware of the signs and symptoms that demonstrate a change in blood glucose level—irritability, argumentative, and sweaty palms.

Table 8.1 Types of diabetes mellitus

Type 1	• Insulin is not produced by the body • Usually appears before the age of 40 years • Least common of the 2 types
Type 2	• Too little insulin produced or insulin is ineffective • Usually linked with obesity • Generally appears after 40 years • Is more prevalent in South Asian and Afro-Caribbean communities • 85% of people with diabetes have type 2

Rheumatic fever

Rheumatic fever is a disease caused by the *Streptococcus* bacteria; it often follows a sore throat. The main concern is the damage that often occurs from fibrosis (stiffening) and distortion of the heart valves. The damage results from inflammation caused by immunological-mediated tissue injury. The disease is now rare in the UK, affecting <0.01% of children.

Signs and symptoms

Acute
- Predominantly affects children aged 5–15 years.
- Sore throat followed by febrile illness (fever).
- Pain moving from joint to joint (giving the disease its name).
- *Streptococcus* bacteria detected in blood samples.
- Chronic damage to heart valves.
- Severe cases have myocarditis (inflammation of the heart muscle).

Chronic
- The heart valve most commonly damaged is the mitral valve (70%), followed by aortic valve (20%).
- A heart murmur can be heard because of damage to heart valves.
- ECG changes.
- Risk of endocarditis.

Treatment

Patients are rarely seen in the acute phase. Medical practitioners prescribe prompt antimicrobial therapy.

Dental implications

- In the acute phase, patients needing emergency dental treatment, such as tooth extraction, should have this carried out under local anaesthesia. General anaesthetic should be avoided because of the possibility of myocarditis.
- No other precautions are necessary.
- Antibiotic prophylaxis to prevent endocarditis is no longer recommended.
- There is no research showing a link between dentistry and endocarditis.
- Fewer patients are harmed by dental treatment without antimicrobial therapy than allergy to the antibiotics prescribed.

Heart-valve replacement

Heart-valve replacement surgery involves implanting either a mechanical or a biological heart valve.

Mechanical valves

These are made from carbon fibre. Sometimes the valves click in operation. Mechanical valves last a long time, usually for life, but they carry a higher risk of causing blood clots. Anticoagulants (blood-thinning drugs) are needed for life.

Biological valves

These are made from human or animal tissue. These valves do not require long-term anticoagulants. Biological valves have a shorter working life and often require a further operation for replacement. Biological valves are not suitable for everyone and are sometimes rejected for personal or religious reasons.

Dental implications

- Many patients take anticoagulants and ∴ extra caution is required for invasive surgical treatments.
- If the patient is taking warfarin, record the international normalized ratio (INR), which measures how soon blood will clot.
- A decision for treatment can now be safely made.

Endocarditis

Endocarditis is the inflammation and thickening of the lining of the heart and predominantly affects the heart valves. Almost any type of heart lesion is susceptible to infection, especially if there is a disturbance in blood flow.

Signs and symptoms

- Can cause coarctation (narrowing) of the aorta.
- Causes progressive heart damage.
- Many organs are affected by embolism (loose clot or debris) from the damaged heart.
- Predisposed by either cardiac damage or bacteraemia (bacteria in the blood).
- The most common microbe isolated is *Streptococcus viridans*—these microbes are dentally related.

Dental implications

- Patients who are susceptible to infective endocarditis should have regular dental check-ups, oral-hygiene instruction, and reinforcement.
- There is no current research evidence to show that endocarditis is caused by dental treatment.

Haemorrhagic problems

The blood consists, in simple terms, of red cells (erythrocytes), white cells (leucocytes), and platelets. Disorders affecting platelets mainly cause haemorrhagic (bleeding) problems, whereas problems with red and white cells are rarer causes of bleeding.

Signs and symptoms

A platelet disorder might present as a nosebleed, bruising on the skin, or bleeding gums that are unrelated to severe gum disease (periodontitis).

Causes of poor blood clotting include the following:
- Haemophilia—a congenital disease, usually affecting ♂:
  - Type A is a deficiency or ↓ in the production of factor VIII, which is needed for blood clotting.
  - Type B is a deficiency in factor IX.
- Von Willebrand's disease—a combined disease because it involves platelets and factor VIII, which affects both ♂ and ♀.
- Thrombocytopenia—failed platelet production.
- Leukaemia.
- Immunological disease, such as HIV.
- Severe liver disease.
- Anticoagulant therapy.

Treatment

Treatment of these conditions is carried out at specialist centres only.

Dental implications

- Patients who have complex clotting problems, such as haemophilia and thrombocytopenia, must be treated in specialist centres. The treatment often requires liaison with specialist haematologists.
- Treatment should be as minimally invasive and atraumatic as possible.
- Treatment should, if possible, be planned well in advance and have a good prognosis for success.
- Adult patients with haemorrhagic problems of this type will usually be under the care of a specialist and often carry a warning card.
- Dentistry can sometimes be the first time a patient is aware of a bleeding disorder, following dental surgery and a slow clotting time.
- Patients on anticoagulants, such as aspirin, warfarin, heparin, and clopidogrel, will require a blood analysis before dental surgery to safely plan the procedure.

Prosthetic replacements

Reasons for prosthetic replacements

A prosthetic replacement is an artificial substitute for a body part that no longer functions and is a hindrance or hazard to the patient. Some prosthetic replacements can be vital for maintaining life, such as heart valves, or the patient's self-esteem, such as an artificial eye or hand.

Invisible prosthetic replacements

Some patients will have prosthetic replacements that are termed 'invisible' and would not be obvious without them disclosing their use. An example would be a person who has suffered breast cancer that required surgical removal of the whole breast tissue. This might then be repaired either with plastic surgery or by wearing prosthetics. This would indicate that the patient has been severely ill and might still be on therapy but, without being told, the dental clinician might never know.

Functions of prosthetic replacements

Prosthetic replacements serve many purposes. Some improve function, others improve appearance, and some improve both function and appearance (e.g. false teeth [dentures], crowns, and bridges). It is important to know that the prosthetic replacement will indeed aid the patient but can never be as good as a perfect body part.

Dental implications

The patient has a prosthetic appliance for a reason and dental staff must be sensitive to the fact that it is worn or fitted for a purpose, which the patient might not always want to reveal. The hidden problems a patient might have could be as follows:
- Physical problems, such as alopecia—the patient wears a wig.
- Psychological problems, such as the patient does not feel like a 'whole person' without the prosthesis.
- Functional problems, e.g. without the prosthesis the patient would die.
- Practical problems, such as the prosthesis helps the patient to manage daily life—an artificial limb.

Dental prostheses provide the patient with an appliance that looks good, restores self-esteem, enables the person to chew their food better, and often halts damage to surrounding teeth, such as overeruption and tilting of opposing and adjacent teeth.

Drug misuse

People misuse drugs because of an addiction to either prescribed or illicit drugs. Patients who visit the dental surgery will not always disclose their addictions because of embarrassment and/or stigma. Individuals who have these addictions sometimes feel that they do not deserve the compassion and understanding given to people with other medical problems, as they perceive that their problems are self-inflicted and 'brought upon themselves'.

Treatment

Treatment might include the following:
- Cognitive behavioural therapy—people are shown the damage that their addiction can do.
- Chemical therapy—people are given medicines that assist them to cope with withdrawal, such as nicotine patches, methadone, and antiemetics (antinausea drugs).
- A personal desire and self-determination to be free of the addiction.

Dental implications

- Patients attending the dental surgery and who have a drug habit often have other complications, such as being heavy smokers and drinkers. They are more prone to oral cancer and often have periodontal problems associated with their habit.
- Alcoholism is associated with cirrhosis, leading to iron deficiency, bleeding problems, and poor metabolism of medicines and drugs.
- People who have an illicit drug habit very often take poor care of their teeth—teeth are low on the scale of importance in their lives. Some of the drugs are given in sugary bases to make them more palatable, even methadone, which is given to people trying to break their drug habit. People who misuse drugs are poor dental attenders and have erratic lifestyles. This can mean that treatment plans requiring a series of subsequent visits are not suitable for these patients.
- The clinician must be aware of the drugs that the patient is taking because there might be an interaction with other medicines that might be prescribed or administered during a course of treatment.

The immunocompromised patient

Patients who are immunocompromised cannot resist infections in the normal manner. This is because of suppression of the immune system, which means that the patient is more prone to infection. Such patients have a medical condition that is being treated but the treatment allows other bacteria or fungi to flourish when the normal environment is altered. This can lead to the patient experiencing various changes, such as oral thrush (a white fungus in the mouth), diarrhoea, and, in the worst cases, death can occur from lung infections from organisms that would not normally be life threatening.

Immunodeficiency can have 2 causes, as outlined here.

Congenital immunodeficiency

A collective term for various different inherited immunodeficiencies which includes deficiency of IgA or IgG (immunoglobulins found in the blood). These immunoglobulins help protect the body and fight infection.

Acquired immunodeficiency

Includes:
- Autoimmune conditions such as coeliac disease, lupus erythematosus, rheumatoid arthritis, and Sjögren's syndrome.
- Diabetes mellitus.
- Infections, such as TB and HIV.
- Neoplasms, such as leukaemia and other cancers.
- Drug therapy—some medicines are designed to suppress the immune response, such as anticancer medicines and corticosteroids.

Dental implications

Patients who are immunocompromised are more likely to acquire infections than other healthy individuals. ▶ It is ∴ very important that cross-infection control in the dental surgery is carried out to the highest standard. Not all procedures in the dental surgery are sterile procedures, but, in some cases, they are considered to be clinically clean. Patients known to be immunocompromised should be protected from further infection by ensuring that, where possible, the treatment carries a low risk of microbial transfer.

Patients with HIV

The largest group of people classified as immunocompromised are those who have HIV. These patients can often be infected by the virus for some time without any signs or symptoms. The dentist is often among the first healthcare workers to be alerted to the patient's condition. The patient would attend the clinic for a dental check-up and the clinician would see oral candida (thrush), angular chelitis (stomatitis), repetitive cold sores, and hairy leucoplakia (white patches). In late cases, the clinician could find Kaposi's sarcoma (a strawberry-red tumour found in the oral cavity), swollen lymph nodes, and sudden weight loss (giving the patient a gaunt and waxy appearance).

People who are living with HIV can receive medication and drug therapy to slow the progression of the disease to acquired immunodeficiency syndrome (AIDS).

These medicines have powerful actions at a cellular and genetic level and will have many side effects, including nausea, diarrhoea, and lipodystrophy (storage of body fat in unusual areas). They can often interact with medicines that the clinician would prescribe for infection or sedation. A full and comprehensive medical history is very important.

The patient is also living with the knowledge that there is currently no cure for this disease. The team should be aware of the psychological difficulties that this must bring.

The child patient

Definition

A person <16 years of age is generally referred to as a child. This is a legal term that has been adopted by the medical and dental professions. Some children mature very quickly and can be considered older and able to make life decisions at <16 years of age, whereas others >16 years of age are still quite childish. The importance of defining an upper age is to decide at what age a patient can give informed consent and does not require the approval of a parent or guardian.

Disadvantages of young age for dentistry

Children have specific problems associated with them, so much so that there are branches of medicine and dentistry specializing in paediatric care (care of children) (see Chapter 15).

Dentition

Children have a 1° set of teeth that usually begin to erupt (show in the mouth) from ~6 months of age. By the age of 2.5 years, 20 1° teeth are in place. The first teeth to be exfoliated (naturally lost) are the lower first 1° incisors. This loss of teeth and their replacement by 2° teeth continues through the mixed dentition, until the age of ~12 years, at which time all 28 permanent teeth have usually erupted.

Dental implications

- Children have fears and anxieties about dentistry that cannot always be explained as easily as to an adult.
- They have a shorter attention span which requires more interpersonal skills and very good clinical skills to complete tasks accurately and swiftly.
- Children's 1° teeth have a different morphology (shape) and the pulp (blood supply and nerve) is encased by a structure in which the enamel is thinner compared with permanent teeth. The pulp horns are also larger.
- Children are prone to accidents, such as falls, and ∴ can damage teeth while they are still developing.
- They can require orthodontic intervention (braces) to correct malaligned (crooked) teeth.
- Dental treatment can include pulpotomies, stainless steel crowns, and the replacement of luxated teeth.
- They are, in unfortunate circumstances, sometimes mistreated by others and can suffer from non-accidental injury.

The older patient

Definition

There are currently >11 million people over retirement age (65 years for ♂ and 60 years for ♀) living in the UK. Furthermore, >1 million people are aged 85 years or more.

Becoming older is an unavoidable fact of life. People could be considered older when they have reached a certain age, such as 70 years. This is termed as 'chronologically old'. Sometimes people seem older because certain circumstances in their life have aged them (e.g. illness and disability). This is termed as 'physiologically old'.

Disadvantages of old age for dentistry

Older people have particular problems associated with ageing. For this reason, specialist medicine and dedicated dental services have been developed, which are called 'geriatric medicine' and 'geriodontology', respectively. The older person often has greater levels of sickness because of organs beginning to fail and joints wearing out. They are slower moving around and take longer to see and treat. Medicines and drugs are prescribed at lower doses, because they are slower to metabolize in the liver.

The older patient can have the following:
- Dementia.
- Parkinson's disease.
- Stroke.
- Angina.
- Respiratory disease.
- Muscle and joint wastage and damage.
- Osteoporosis.
- Age-related deafness and eyesight problems.
- Poor oral health.
- Poor diet.

Dental implications

- A good medical history is essential if the patient is to be treated safely. It is wise to be aware of what medicines the older person is taking, such as warfarin, GTN, and bisphosphonates.
- The older person is usually taking several medicines prescribed by the GP.
- The dental team must be sympathetic to the speed that a patient can access the surgery and angle at which they can be treated.
- Dentistry must be easily carried out, give a good prognosis, and be easily maintained.
- Many patients are less dextrous and cannot look after their teeth as well as they could when they were younger.
- Many medicines are taken for underlying medical conditions and these cause xerostomia (dry mouth), which leads to dental decay. Cervical caries (tooth decay of the root) is very difficult to treat.
- Some patients cannot receive and retain information, so it is prudent to have a carer or escort with them at the dental visit.

- Mobility difficulties might include the use of walking sticks, frames, and wheelchairs.
- Prostheses might be worn, such as glasses, hearing aids, wigs, and false teeth, all of which can make dental treatment more difficult.
- Skin is more delicate in the older patient, so it is important for the nurse to make sure that the aspirator etc. does not rub too heavily on the skin, which can easily become sore/cracked.

The disabled patient

Definition
The World Health Organization (WHO) definition of disability is 3-fold and divided into 3 main terms:[1]
- Impairment—any loss or abnormality of psychological, physiological, or anatomical structure or function.
- Disability—any restriction or lack of ability to perform an activity in the manner, or within the range, considered normal for a human being (as a result of an impairment).
- Handicap—a function of the relationship between disabled persons and their environment caused by the loss of opportunities to take part in the life of the community on an equal level with others.

The disabled patient can be any age and the disability might be congenital or acquired.

Disadvantages of disability for dentistry
Patients who are born with a disability or have the disability from an early age will often cope better with the difficulty compared with someone who has acquired the disability later in life—e.g. it is more difficult for a patient who has accidental spinal injury to cope with a wheelchair than someone who has used it from a very early age.

There are 6.5 million people with disabilities in UK.

Dental example
- Impairment—loss of a front tooth.
- Disability—unable to eat some foods.
- Handicap—unable to go out socially for a meal.

Legal requirements
People with disabilities are now protected by law—the Disabled Discrimination Act (1995 and 2005). People with disabilities have the right to the following:
- Employment.
- Education.
- Access to goods, facilities, and services.
- Buying or renting land or property.

Dental implications
- People with disabilities have more social difficulties.
- The more visible a disability is to another person, the easier it is for them to obtain appropriate treatment.
- It is not easy to obtain routine dental care if access to the clinic is difficult.
- Some obvious impairments have hidden ones, such as paraplegia and incontinence.
- Some people with disabilities feel stigmatized as being difficult to treat, a nuisance, and demanding.

- Discuss all treatments with the patient and don't assume that people with disabilities have ↓ cognitive abilities. For example, people with cerebral palsy have difficulty speaking but often have normal intelligence.

[1] World Health Organization (1980). *International classification of impairments, disabilities and handicaps: a manual of classification relating to the consequences of disease.* Geneva: WHO.

The anxious patient

Definition

Anxiety is a vague, unpleasant feeling accompanied by the thought that something undesirable is about to happen. It can occur in response to a specific stimulus.

Fear of the dentist is not uncommon. Research has shown that, in most cases, dental anxiety stems from an earlier bad experience at the dentist. The patient might be anxious because they are nervous and anxious by nature. Some people are anxious and cautious about 'life' in general. They are concerned about various life experiences, such as flying, new environments, and trying unusual food.

Some people are anxious after hearing of other people's negative experiences at the dentist.

Recognizing anxiety

Staff will often spot an anxious patient when they first arrive for an appointment, as follows:
- Facial and body language.
- Inappropriate laughter or sharpness of responses.
- Sweaty lip and hands.
- Pallor.
- The patient might be upfront and tell you about the anxiety.

Dental staff should take the patient's concerns very seriously, because a patient who feels that they are being listened to and not treated as a nuisance or someone who is making a fuss over nothing will form a trust more readily. Showing a patient empathy improves the communication pathway, as follows:
- ↑ patient satisfaction.
- ↑ patient compliance.
- ↓ anxiety.
- ↑ dental team–patient rapport.
- ↑ dental team–patient satisfaction.
- ↓ team stress.

Dental implications

- Patients may avoid appointments.
- The initial reason for dental anxiety is often quite different from that which keeps it going.

The patient requiring special care

Definition

Patients can sometimes be referred to as having 'special needs'. This is an outdated term and is no longer considered acceptable. The person requires special care but has exactly the same needs as you and me.

Special-care dentistry covers treatment of the following:
- Learning disability.
- Drug and alcohol misuse.
- Medically compromised patients.
- Physically disabled.
- Mental health.
- Older people.
- Anxious or phobic people.

Disadvantages

This category of patient will require longer to treat or a specialized knowledge of the problem to either improve the patient's experience or keep the patient safe throughout the treatment.

There are often communication difficulties, which includes communicating with the following people:
- Patient.
- Carer/guardian/escort/advocate.
- Doctor—general medical practitioner.
- Specialist nurse/physician.
- Residential care home.
- Medical/dental protection society.
- Independent mental capacity advocate (IMCA).

Dental implications

Special-care dentistry might require the need for the following:
- Special drugs or medicines and/or care with drug interactions.
- Special access, such as wider door entry, use of a hoist, and use of a wheelchair tipper or transfer.
- Coordinated care with other disciplines, such as working alongside an anaesthetist or haematologist.
- Use of adapted equipment, such as a toothbrush with a big-grip handle and mouth guards.
- Use of sedation or general anaesthesia.

Dental nurses can specialize after qualification through the NEBDN Special Care Dentistry course.

Social, cultural, and psychological constraints

The UK population is made up of a diverse range of individuals. This diversity brings with it differences in social, cultural, and religious considerations for the dental practice.

Social and cultural constraints

Social and cultural differences are demonstrated in many ways, such as when ♀ from some ethnic backgrounds prefer to be treated by ♀ practitioners or a ♂ dentist is not expected to shake the hand of a ♀ patient.

Some people have strict religious constraints that allow treatment only on certain days or times. A Jewish patient cannot have treatment on a Friday evening or Saturday. Furthermore, a Muslim patient might not be able to have dental treatment during Ramadan because they would prefer not to have water (used a lot in dentistry) in the mouth at this time. Some patients refuse some treatments because they are made from or use 'unclean', non-kosher, or other unsuitable sources.

Psychological constraints

Some people have psychological constraints that prevent them from accepting routine dental treatment. This might be because of personal beliefs (e.g. amalgam is a dangerous material in teeth that causes neurological problems because of the mercury content).

Communication

Defining communication

What is communication?

Communication is the process of exchanging information. The person giving the information first thinks about what information must be transferred and then sends that information to the other person. That person accepts the information, processes it, and responds and the cycle continues.

Why is communication important?

In the dental environment, communication is very important. Patients must receive accurate and high-quality information to enable them to make an informed decision on dental treatment. If the information given is unclear, a patient could become confused about the treatment being offered, which could lead to treatment the patient later regrets. If a patient does not fully understand the information, they cannot give informed consent, which in turn has legal implications. Good communication between members of the dental team is also of great importance. Team members should be able to communicate information to each other so that they can work together effectively and provide a high standard of care for their patients.

What factors affect communication?

Lots of things can affect the way that communication takes place. The way you look, the body language you use, your tone, and the level of your voice can all have an effect on how the receiver interprets the information. The language that you use can have a key role in communicating information to patients, especially in explaining treatment procedures. All dental professionals spend a great deal of their training course learning the correct terminology in relation to dentistry, but the terminology can be confusing for the patient.

▶ Do not use jargon or abbreviations when giving information to patients because some individuals might be too embarrassed to ask for further explanations.

Methods of communication

Communication can be verbal or non-verbal, or a combination of both.

Verbal communication

There are thousands of different languages and dialects spoken across the world, so it is no surprise that speech is the most used form of communication. Although you may speak the same language, the development of slang, age, gender, social class, profession, and other factors might have an effect on understanding. For example, a simple sentence, such as 'an RDN is a DCP who is registered with the GDC and must do regular CPD', might make perfect sense to a qualified dental nurse but could sound confusing to a hairdresser.

▶ When communicating information to patients, try to explain using language that they will understand and ask them if they have any questions so you can clarify any issues for them. Consider the tone and pace (how quickly or slowly you speak) so that the patient feels at ease.

Non-verbal communication

This type of communication can complement or hinder verbal communication. Thoughts and feelings can often be expressed by use of body language or facial expressions, by either the giver or the receiver of the information. How many times have you raised your eyebrows when being told something, started to smile as you are saying something comical, or frowned when being told something that is confusing or you don't believe? Think back to when you were a child and would instantly know you were in trouble by the look given to you by one of your parents.

Body language

Body language plays a huge part in communication and affects how individuals interact. As a dental nurse, you will be required to monitor your patient during treatment, which involves observing their behaviour. Certain actions they make can indicate whether they are feeling nervous or anxious about their treatment (e.g. fidgeting, arms crossed, speaking a lot, or not speaking very much at all) and much of this is non-verbal. You can use your body language to reassure patients, such as making eye contact with them and smiling when they enter the clinical area rather than not looking at them and appearing solemn. Using eye contact can give the impression that you are listening/interested in what someone is communicating to you. However, do not stare continually because this can make the other person very uncomfortable or make you seem aggressive! Be aware of the body language you use when a patient is talking to you. Show you are listening by making eye contact, leaning (only slightly) towards them, and nodding in agreement.

Body position

Body position and posture are also important. Think of your position and posture when you are talking to family and friends and how they would differ if you were talking to another medical professional. Keep a comfortable distance when talking to patients and try not to invade their personal space, but remember the rules of personal space change when you assist with treatment.

Gestures

Gestures with hands/arms can be used when explaining but try not to be too elaborate or you might seem to be flapping about and this can be distracting for both parties.

Clothing

Appearance can have an effect on how we might act and how others perceive us. Everybody has their own perception of how professional people should appear. From a patient's point of view, how would you feel if you went to see your doctor and they had just thrown on an old pair of jeans and unironed t-shirt, with unbrushed hair? Would you feel differently if they were dressed smartly and had a tidy appearance? Now think of how you feel when you are dressed in your uniform for work and when you have just put on any old thing to slob around they house in. If you are correctly dressed in your uniform, you will be seen and treated as a professional.

Written information

Signs, symbols, and written information can also be given in addition to verbal communication. Make sure written information is clear and concise, can be easily understood, and is in line with the verbal information being given.

▶ There is nothing worse than being told one thing and given written instructions that contradict what was given verbally.

Touch

There are times when a patient might find touch reassuring and offering a hand for them to hold or placing a hand on their shoulder or arm can help put them at ease. Touch should not be used just because you feel the patient needs it; e.g. if the patient is having a complex surgical extraction and is apparently at ease but you feel the procedure is complex and try to reassure the patient through touch, this could unnerve the patient because they might think 'is everything ok or is the treatment going badly?'

Barriers to communication

There are many reasons why communication could fail to develop or break down. Being aware of these can help you identify when you might need to take different approaches to communication or seek further help. Some of the common barriers are outlined in this section.

Language/culture

One of the most common communication differences is a language barrier. This might be as straightforward as 2 people speaking different languages or it could result from different accents or cultural differences.

Language

Translators can be used if there is a difference in language but they should be experienced in translating dental treatments and terminology because some words don't exist in other languages and ∴ need further explanation. Family members or children should not be used as translators because there is no guarantee they are translating the information accurately to the patient.

Culture

Sometimes a patient's culture might affect the process of communication. Some cultures don't deem it appropriate for ♀ to talk directly to ♂ so a ♀'s father, brother, or husband might speak for them.

Environment

The environment can affect the way in which people communicate. A patient might feel uneasy or nervous in the dental environment and not be as easy to communicate with; that is, it might be difficult to get information from them. However, this has an opposite effect on some people and they might feel they need to tell you everything.

Gender

There are some things that people find difficult talking to the opposite sex about. This can be especially evident when it comes to discussing medical histories or personal issues.

Appearance

A person's appearance can often have an effect on how others communicate with them. For example, someone in a professional uniform might be spoken to in a more professional manner than someone wearing jeans and a tee-shirt. Imagine how you expect members of certain professions (e.g. policemen, nurses, and doctors) to look. Sometimes people can experience what is referred to as 'white-coat syndrome' or 'white-coat hypertension', which is caused by the anxiety felt by a person in a clinical/medical environment.

Physical disabilities

These can be anything from partial or total blindness or deafness, or a combination of both. These disabilities will require communication with care; for example, it's no good asking a blind patient to follow you into the surgery or calling out to a deaf person if they can't see you.

General barriers to avoid

Certain behaviours can have a negative effect on communication. Some common examples to avoid are as follows:

- Appearing bored or impatient.
- Using abusive or threatening language.
- Challenging behaviour.
- Not paying attention to the other person.
- Mumbling or not speaking clearly.
- Interrupting or finishing sentences.
- Jumping to conclusions.
- Being judgemental.
- Being in a distracting environment.

To improve communication, remember to do the following:

- Think about what you say before you say it.
- Speak clearly, without using jargon.
- Listen carefully to what is being said.
- Think about what is said before you reply.
- Ask questions to clarify any information.

Assessment of oral health needs and treatment

Record keeping

▶ The importance of good, accurate record keeping cannot be emphasized enough. In the event of a patient making a complaint or an allegation against a member of the dental team the clinical records may be vital.

What should be recorded?

Records should contain facts and state the treatment that has taken place. Patients refusing treatment and failed or cancelled appointments should also be recorded in the notes.

Detrimental comments should be avoided.

How long should records be retained?

- For adults, patient notes, X-rays, and models must be stored for 11 years.
- For children, records should be stored until the patient reaches 25 years of age or for 11 years, whichever occurs first.

Retrieving records

Should a patient make a complaint, contact your appropriate defence organization. Keep all original documentation in a safe place—never send original documentation, always make copies. Advice should be sought on litigation matters as soon as possible.

National Health Service (NHS) charting in the UK

A method of dental charting has been developed that can easily be recognized and understood by all dental professionals. The system is a quick and easy way to record the dentition of an individual:

Orientation of the chart

The mouth is divided into 4 quadrants
- Upper right.
- Upper left.
- Lower right.
- Lower left.

Individual teeth in each quadrant are then identified according to their surfaces:
- Molar and premolar teeth are divided into the occlusal, mesial, distal, palatal/lingual, and buccal/labial surfaces.
- Incisors and canines are divided into mesial, distal, palatal/lingual, and buccal/labial surfaces with an incisal edge or canine cusp.

Numbering system

Each quadrant starts at the midline and finishes at the 3rd molar tooth. The permanent dentition is represented by the numbers 1–8 and deciduous dentition is represented by the letters a–e. Each tooth is referred to by its quadrant and number, as the following examples show:
- Upper right permanent central incisor—UR1.
- Lower left permanent 3rd molar—LL8.
- Lower left deciduous central incisor—LLa.

Examination procedure

The examination is carried out using a dental mouth mirror and probe. The mouth mirror is used to facilitate the dentist's view and a straight probe is used to examine the hard tissues (teeth). A Briault probe enables the dentist to examine the interproximal areas of the teeth (see Appendix, Fig. A.7).

Using the chart

The condition of the teeth is noted on the chart and restorations can be charted by the use of recognized notations (see 📖 Accepted notations, p.228 and Fig. 10.1).

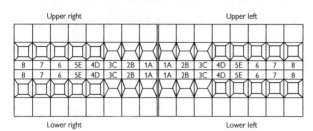

Fig. 10.1 A typical teeth numbering chart used in the UK. Reproduced with permission from NEBDN.

International Dental Federation (FDI) charting

The FDI charting system of 'notation' or 'teeth numbering charts' is similar to the NHS system in the UK, with the exception of the way the teeth are identified.

Teeth are still divided into quadrants, but the quadrants are numbered and deciduous teeth are given a number rather than a letter.

Permanent dentition

See Fig. 10.2.
- Upper right—quadrant 1.
- Upper left—quadrant 2.
- Lower left—quadrant 3.
- Lower right—quadrant 4.

Deciduous dentition

See Fig. 10.3.
- Upper right—quadrant 5.
- Upper left—quadrant 6.
- Lower left—quadrant 7.
- Lower right—quadrant 8.

Numbering system

Each tooth is referred to by its quadrant and number, as the following examples show:
- Upper right permanent central incisor—11
- Lower left permanent 3rd molar—38.
- Lower right deciduous canine—83.
- Upper left deciduous 1st molar—64.

Permanent dentition	
Upper right Quadrant 1	Upper left Quadrant 2
Lower right Quadrant 4	Lower left Quadrant 3

18 17 16 15 14 13 12 11	21 22 23 24 25 26 27 28
48 47 46 45 44 43 42 41	31 32 33 34 35 36 37 38

Fig. 10.2 FDI quadrant numbering for the permanent dentition. Reproduced with permission from NEBDN.

Deciduous dentition	
Upper right Quadrant 5	Upper left Quadrant 6
Lower right Quadrant 8	Lower left Quadrant 7

55 54 53 52 51	61 62 63 64 65
85 84 83 82 81	71 72 73 74 75

Fig. 10.3 FDI quadrant numbering for the deciduous dentition. Reproduced with permission from NEBDN.

Basic periodontal examination (BPE) charting

Periodontal disease is quite often painless and can remain undetected for many years unless a thorough examination is carried out (see 📖 Periodontal diseases, p.143). A system has been developed to quickly and clearly note the presence of periodontal disease.

Examination procedure

A BPE is carried out to assess the condition of the patient's soft tissues. The mouth is divided into sextants (Fig. 10.4) and the presence of periodontal pockets is recorded onto a chart (Fig. 10.5).

Periodontal pockets are measured by use of a BPE/Community Periodontal Index of Treatment Needs (CPITN) probe and each pocket is given a score, depending on its condition.

BPE scores

The higher the code, the more serious the periodontal disease (Table 10.1). Patients presenting with a score of 3, 4, or * require their individual pocket depths to be recorded in full so that intensive periodontal treatment can be initiated.

Upper teeth

Teeth 8–4	Teeth 3–3	Teeth 4–8
Teeth 8–4	Teeth 3–3	Teeth 4–8

Lower teeth

Fig. 10.4 BPE sextants within the mouth.

1	2	1
2	2	2

Fig. 10.5 Example of a completed chart.

Table 10.1 BPE scores

Code	Condition of the pocket
0	Healthy gingival tissues, no bleeding
1	Coloured area of the probe is visible; no calculus present; no defective margins present; bleeding on probing; pocket depth <3.5mm
2	Coloured area of the probe is visible; plaque retention factors detected; pocket depth <3.5mm
3	Coloured area of the probe is partly visible; pocket depth <5.5mm
4	Coloured area of the probe is not visible; pocket depth >6mm
*	Involvement of the furcation or recession; pocket depth ≥7mm

Full periodontal assessment

A full periodontal assessment is carried out to record the mobility, plaque retention, bleeding, and pocket depth of each individual tooth and its surrounding gingival.

Examination procedure

Pocket depths are measured by use of a periodontal probe that is graduated in millimeters (see 📖 Basic periodontal examination (BPE), p.156). The results of the assessment are recorded onto a periodontal chart (Fig. 10.6).

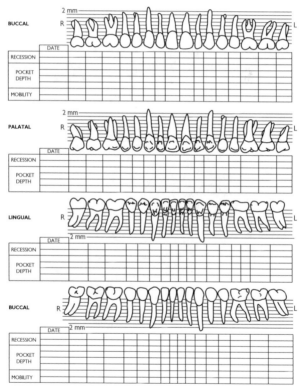

Fig. 10.6 Periodontal examination chart. Reproduced with permission from NEBDN.

Accepted notations

There are various notations that can be used in dental charting and many dentists have their own preferred methods and symbols. However, the National Examining Board for Dental Nurses (NEBDN) has developed a national standard that is easy to use and recognize by dental professionals.

Using the chart

A standard NHS chart is normally used to record teeth present, existing restorations, and missing teeth on the central line of boxes. Any work that must be carried out is recorded in the outer line of boxes (see Fig. 10.7 and ☐ National Health Service (NHS) charting in the UK, p.222).

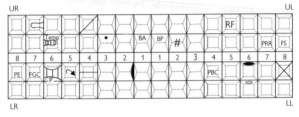

Fig. 10.7 Example of a completed chart. Reproduced with permission from NEBDN.

Study models

A laboratory needs a model of the patient's jaw to make a removable prostheses or orthodontic appliance.

Making study models

Models are constructed from an impression of the patient's mouth that is taken by the dentist and sent to the laboratory. At the laboratory, the technician pours plaster into the impression of the patient's jaw. When set, the plaster model forms a replica of the patient's jaw that the technician can use to construct the prostheses or appliance.

For some procedures, the technician will need to know the patient's jaw relationship. This is recorded by the dentist by use of occlusal rims. The rims are returned to the laboratory, where the technician uses them to set the models onto an articulator. An articulator is a hinged mechanism that keeps models in the correct relationship.

Recording progress by use of study models

For orthodontic treatment, study (record) models are made before, during, and after treatment. Models made before treatment is carried out are used to decide on the plan of treatment. Further models are taken during treatment to record progress and final models are taken to monitor the end result. To enable the dental technician to prepare models in the correct occlusion (biting position), a squash bite can be taken from the patient. The dentist takes a squash bite by use of a piece of softened modelling wax. The patient is asked to bite down on the wax so that the occlusion is recorded and this is sent to the laboratory.

Patient charges and exemptions

A NHS dentist is one who has agreed with their primary care trust (PCT) to provide NHS dental care services to their local community.

NHS charges in the UK

There are 3 standard charges for patients who pay for their treatment: the amount paid depends on the treatment needed to maintain healthy teeth and gums. The bands are as follows:

- Band 1—examination, diagnosis (x-rays), scaling, and polishing (if needed), and advice on how to prevent further oral health problems.
- Band 2—items listed in band 1 plus any further treatment, such as fillings, root canal treatment, and extractions.
- Band 3—items covered in bands 1 and 2 plus crowns, dentures, or bridges.

Costs

The charge for each band is set by the NHS and reviewed annually.[1] Charges set in April 2011 are as follows:

- Band 1—£17.
- Band 2—£47.
- Band 3—£204.

Private charges

Several dental treatments, such as white fillings on occlusal surfaces of posterior teeth and gold crowns on anterior teeth, are not available on the NHS. A patient may ∴ choose to have some of their dental treatment carried out privately. A dentist who provides private dental treatment will have their own set charges for individual items.

Before any dental treatment is carried out, patients should be made aware of their treatment options and what can be provided on the NHS or privately. They should be told how much their treatment will cost and given a written treatment plan (including costs). This should be kept with the patient records.

Exemptions

A patient is eligible for free NHS dental treatment if they qualify under any of the following criteria when treatment starts:

- Aged <18 years of age.
- Aged >18 years of age and in full-time education.
- Pregnant or have a baby <12 months of age.
- An NHS inpatient when treatment is carried out by a hospital dentist.
- An NHS hospital dental service outpatient.
- The patient or their partner receives income support, income-based jobseekers allowance, or pension guarantee credit.
- Entitled to, or named on, a valid NHS tax credit exemption certificate.
- Named on a HC2 certificate which entitles the named individual to free dental treatment along with additional benefits.

---

[1] http://www.nhs.uk/nhsengland/aboutnhsservices/dentists/pages/nhs-dental-treatments.aspx.

Dental radiography

Radiation

Radiation cannot be seen, smelt, heard, or felt and is ∴ difficult to detect. In minute quantities radiation can be considered harmless, but excessive exposure to radiation can be hazardous and ∴ should not be ignored. Most people have been exposed to radiation in the form of a dental or medical x-ray. This form of radiation is known as 'electromagnetic' and not only includes x-rays, but also includes gamma (γ)-rays. When a photographic type film is exposed to x-rays and developed, it will produce an image, depending on what the x-rays passed through before reaching the film. This image is known as a radiograph.

An overdose of radiation can cause undesirable side effects that range from mild burns to leukaemia, depending on the dose administered.

Uses

X-rays are used in dentistry for many reasons. They can aid diagnosis and support treatment planning for individual patients. Depending on the type of film used, radiographs will show the following:
- Unerupted teeth, impacted teeth, and retained roots in either the upper or the lower jaw.
- Tooth and root morphology, especially in relation to shape, size, and the number of roots of each individual tooth.
- Surrounding alveolar bone.
- A chronic alveolar abscess around the apex of a non-vital tooth.
- Progression during endodontic treatment, including diagnostic working length, placement of master gutta-percha point, and final restoration.
- Detection of dental caries within the dentition.
- Development of the dentition in relation to developing teeth in a child and for orthodontic assessment.
- Detection of fractures, cysts.

Radiation safety

To ensure that all members of the dental team, patients, and visitors are best protected, the principles outlined here should be followed.

Methods of minimizing exposure

- Use of fast film (E speed) will enable the shortest possible exposure time, ∴ ↓ the amount of radiation the patient is exposed to.
- Sets with adjustable apertures must be correctly positioned to emit the narrowest beam of x-rays for the size of film. Unless approved qualifications are held, this should only be undertaken by the dentist.
- Special film holder/beam-aiming devices should be used for periapical and bite-wing radiographs. This, hopefully, will ↓ the need for retakes.
- All dental staff should stand well clear of the beam during exposure. On no account must a nurse hold the film in place for a patient or uncooperative child.
- Every radiograph must be not only necessary, but also of diagnostic value. It is no longer appropriate to take radiographs without a justified reason.
- X-ray sets should be disconnected from their electricity supply when not in use.

Monitoring exposure

The amount of stray radiation received by staff members can be monitored by use of a film badge. This is an intraoral film, which is worn on the chest or waist for up to 3 months. Film badges are called 'personal monitoring dose meters' and supplied by the National Radiological Protection Board (NRPB). The organization processes the films and notifies the practice of the radiation dosage received; they can arrange appropriate investigation if the dosage is too high.

Long-term safety

Radiation safety must be checked at least every 3 years to ensure sets are adequately shielded, preventing stray radiation. This assessment should only be carried out by a qualified individual and never attempted by any member of staff within the dental practice. Records of this inspection should be kept.

Legislation and regulations

Introduction to radiography

Almost every dental patient will have radiographs taken at some stage of their treatment. This might be at the beginning, to help establish what treatment will be needed, or during treatment, e.g. to assist with establishing working lengths during endodontic treatment.

Although it is neither the responsibility nor the role of the dental nurse to take radiographs, a basic knowledge of radiation and radiography is essential.

Radiation is extremely hazardous, which cannot be seen, smelt, heard, or felt. With this in mind, there are regulations that must be followed to ensure the safety and well-being of both the dental staff and the patients visiting the dental surgery.

Ionizing Radiation (Medical Exposure) Regulations 2000

These regulations deal with the protection of the person undergoing the exposure.

The Ionizing Radiations Regulations 1999 (IRR99)

In January 2000, IRR99 came into force, superseding the previous regulations of 1985. These regulations are in place to ensure that those exposed to radiation as part of their work are exposed to as little of it as possible. This approach can be embodied by the terms 'as low as reasonably achievable' (ALARA) and 'as low as reasonably practicable' (ALARP). In this case, the dentist is considered the employer and ∴ has a duty of care to protect their employees from ionizing radiation in the workplace, in addition to protecting the patient.

Maintenance

X-ray machinery should be maintained and tested on a regular basis, according to specific instructions from the company designated to check the machinery. This work should be carried out by a qualified individual from the company, not anyone else. A log book should be kept, indicating the date when the machine was serviced, who it was serviced by, any work that needed to be carried out on the machinery, and the next service date.

Controlled areas

Controlled areas around all x-ray machinery should be clearly marked. All dental staff should be at least 1.5m away from the dental chair when a radiograph is taken. The only persons permitted within this area are the patient and parent or guardian of an uncooperative/difficult child. The dental nurse should not stay in the area with the patient.

Local rules

These should be placed in an appropriate location. Ensure that the following information is available:
- The name of the Radiation Protection Adviser and Radiation Protection Supervisor for the dental surgery.
- A contingency plan in the event of a machinery incident.
- Precautions to take—for both staff members and patients.
- Information relating to the controlled area.

Quality assurance/audit

Audits and quality-assurance procedures should be carried out to ensure that all radiographs are of a high standard, both from a diagnostic/clinical aspect and also in terms of quality of development etc. Such audits are the responsibility of all dental team members involved in the taking and interpretation of radiographs. If problems are identified, they should be assessed and the reason for the failure should be determined. This might lead to training issues, which will need to be addressed.

Radiation protection supervisor (RPS)

An RPS is an individual appointed to ensure that all staff members comply with the regulations. This individual could be any member of the dental team provided they are competent within this field and received appropriate training.

Radiation protection advisor (RPA)

An RPA is an appointed individual who provides advice on IRR99. It is this individual's responsibility to ensure that the regulations are being complied with.

The dentist must ensure that the RPA meets specified criteria in relation to the health and safety executive guidance.

These personnel are externally appointed and offer advice, support, and guidance, as appropriate.

Justification

It is essential to justify why an exposure to ionizing radiation is required, e.g. when the diagnostic working length is required during endodontic treatment. Ensure that doses are also kept to a minimum.

❶ Unless a qualified dental nurse has undergone an approved course of training and met the required standard set by the awarding body, they cannot take radiographs and ∴ should not be put in that position by an insistent dentist.

Techniques and principles

 It is not the role of the dental nurse to position a film in the patient's mouth, set the machine, or position the x-ray tube, unless the appropriate qualifications have been achieved.

To take radiographs you must possess a post-qualification certificate in dental radiography in addition to 1 of the following dental nurse qualifications:
- National Certificate for Dental Nurses.
- The Hospital Diploma in Dental Nursing.
- S/NVQ Level 3 Dental Nurse Certificate.
- Certificate in Higher Education in Dental Nursing.

Basic principles

The electricity supply of the x-ray machine should be switched on. The dentist will confirm the patient's name and reason why the x-ray is required. This should also be documented in the patient's records/notes. Depending on the tooth/teeth being x-rayed and film being used, the correct exposure time will be set on the machine. On newer machines this is usually preset.

When the patient is positioned in the chair, the dentist will place the film in the patient's mouth. The patient might be required to hold the film in place. If not, a film holder should be used. The film is placed in the holder and this, in turn, is positioned in the patient's mouth. Most film holders also have beam-aiming devices that assist the dentist in placing the tube.

The biggest problems encountered when taking x-rays are the risk of the patient moving while the film is being exposed and the x-ray tube being placed incorrectly. It is the responsibility of the dentist, and not the dental nurse, to position both the x-ray film and the tube.

Types of film

There are 2 main types of film used in dental treatment:

Intraoral film

A film taken inside the mouth (see Table 11.1 for the main types of intraoral film).

Table 11.1 The 3 main types of intraoral film

Film type	Uses	Shows
Bite-wing	Detection of interproximal caries	Molars and premolars in occlusion
	Assessment of interproximal alveolar bone	Crest of alveolar bone
		Overhanging restorations
Periapical	Endodontic treatment	Individual tooth and root
	Root fractures	Surrounding alveolar bone
	Chronic alveolar abscess	2–3mm from apex
	Assessment before difficult extraction	
Occlusal	To show unerupted teeth	Plan view of either jaw
	Cysts	

Extraoral film

A film taken outside the mouth (see Table 11.2 for the main types of extraoral film).

Table 11.2 The 3 main types of extraoral film

Film type	Uses	Shows
Panoramic	Unerupted teeth	1 or both sides of both jaws
	Supernumerary teeth	All the teeth
	Fractures of the teeth or jaws	
Lateral cephalometric	Orthodontic treatment planning	Front or side views of the skull
	Jaw surgery	
Lateral oblique	These films unfortunately are considered to have little diagnostic value	Can show position of 3rd molars

Manually processing x-ray films

Most dental practices have either an automatic processor for x-rays or digital radiography facilities. Nevertheless, dental nurses should be aware of how to process films in a manual setting in case the automatic processor becomes unusable. Manual processing is now not that common. However, some surgeries might still have the facilities to carry out manual processing.

Equipment and its preparation

If manual processing is still used, it is probable that the practice will have a dedicated dark room available for processing films. This room is usually quite small but contains a selection of tanks, which sit in another, larger, tank of water, and an immersion heater. This can be heated and ∴ kept at the correct temperature for developing and processing films.

The developing solution is in the 1st tank. This should be covered with a lid to stop the chemicals becoming contaminated. The next tank contains (tap) water, which is used to remove the developing solution on the film. The 3rd tank contains fixing solution and this should also be covered with a lid to prevent contamination from the developing solution. The final tank contains water.

▶ Tanks should be checked daily by the dental nurse to ensure the levels of processing solutions are correct. The water should be changed every day, so this is best done first thing in the morning. The heater can then be switched on to enable the chemicals to warm up.

Chemicals (fixing and developing solutions)

❶ These chemicals are hazardous. Correct PPE should be worn. This will include a pair of safety glasses or a visor, disposable gloves, and a mask.

- The chemicals normally arrive at the dental surgery in large bottles, which must be stored in a locked, fire-proof cupboard to comply with both the Health and Safety at Work Act 1974 and the COSHH Regulations.
- When required, the chemicals are dispensed into separate tanks—1 for the developing solution and 1 for the fixing solution.
- The developing solution is used to develop the image that has been produced, but the image will not stay on the film until it has been fixed into place.
- The fixing solution is used to fix the image on the film.

Temperature

- The ideal temperature is usually 18–22°C. This should be checked by the dental nurse by use of a thermometer. If the temperature is incorrect, it could damage the film (see ▥ Film faults: what went wrong? p.246). The immersion heater can be turned up or down, depending on the temperature required by the manufacturer. The film should not be processed until the correct temperature has been reached.

Lighting
- The dark room will contain 2 lights:
  - A normal light—used initially to check all the chemicals and surrounding area. Any rubbish should be removed to ensure a clean and clear working area.
  - A safe light—normally a red light bulb. This light should be checked for signs of damage. The light should be switched on and the bulb should be checked for possible leaking of white light. If this is the case, the bulb should be changed. If it was left, the film could be exposed to light and ∴ damaged. Normal light would damage an undeveloped film.

Final checks
- Check that all the surfaces are clean, dry, and clear of clutter.
- Place a label with the patient's details on a hanger so that the film can be identified.

Developing films
Preparing to develop the film (under normal lighting)
- Check the manufacturer's instructions on the time the film requires in the developing and fixing solutions.
- Check the temperature of the chemicals by use of a thermometer. The temperatures of the chemicals should be supplied by the manufacturer and these should be checked.
- Ensure that the alarm clock you have is functioning and correct before starting.
- The levels of the chemicals should have been checked first thing in the morning but ensure they are at the correct level before starting. This is normally indicated by a fill line on each individual tank.
- Label a film hanger with the date and patient's name.

Dipping the film into the developing solution (under red lighting)
- Shut the door and lock it from the inside, to prevent anybody entering the room. Light from outside of the developing room will damage the undeveloped film once opened.
- Turn on the safe light and then turn off the main light.
- Allow your eyes to adjust to the light, which can take a few minutes.
- Carefully unwrap the film packet, trying not to bend the film or touch it with your fingers. The film can be found between black papers.
- Place the film on the labelled hanger.
- Remove the lid from the developing solution.
- Holding the top of the hanger with your hand, carefully place the film in the developing solution.
- Set your alarm to the recommended time for the developing solution that is being used.

Removing the film from the developing solution under red lighting

- When the alarm sounds, carefully remove the film from the solution by the top of the hanger. Carefully hold the hanger and attached film over the developing tank to allow excess solution to drip back into the tank and not on to the work surface. Any spillages should be cleaned up as soon as possible to prevent the film possibly becoming damaged later.
- Replace the lid on the tank to prevent contamination.
- Rinse the film under cold running water for 30 seconds.

Dipping the film into the fixing solution under red lighting

- Remove the lid from the fixing solution. Holding the top of the hanger with your hand, carefully place the film in the fixing solution.
- Set your alarm to the recommended time for the fixing solution that is being used.
- When the alarm sounds, remove the film from the fixing solution and allow excess solution to drip back into the tank.
- With the other hand, replace the lid onto the fixing solution. Wash the film again under a flow of running water.

Drying

- It might now be necessary to let the film dry before being mounted. If this is the case, the film can be left on the hanger in a dry area of the dark room—as the film is now fully developed, no special precautions with light are needed.

Automatic and digital processing

Automatic processors

Over the years, and with advancing technologies, automatic processing has become the accepted and easier way to develop films.

Advantages

- Chemicals can be maintained at the correct temperature.
- All films are exposed to the chemicals for the correct time.
- Films go through the appropriate solutions in the correct order.
- Films can be fed through the processor quicker, ∴ more films can be processed.
- Chemicals are enclosed, which minimizes spillage.
- The processor has its own built-in dark area, in which films can be opened without being exposed to light.

Disadvantages

- The automatic machines can be very expensive.
- The processor requires regular cleaning according to the manufacturer's instructions.
- If they break down, you might have to adopt the manual technique of developing films.

Equipment and its preparation

When the machine is dismantled, you will see 3 chambers (sections) within the machine. The 1st chamber will contain the developing solution, the 2nd chamber will contain the fixing solution, and the 3rd chamber will contain water. These chambers should be checked at the start of the day to ensure that the chemicals are at the correct levels. The water should be changed on a daily basis. The machine should then be put back together.

Preparing to develop the film

If the equipment is ready, the dental nurse can switch the automatic processor on and allow time for the chemicals to heat up. Most machines indicate with a light when the chemicals are at the correct temperature. Films should not be placed in the automatic developer until the light has gone out, because the film might be damaged during processing.

When the film has been exposed, it will require developing. Black elastic cuffs are situated on either side of the automatic processor to prevent light leaking in. Small films can be passed through the hand cuffs into the machine, whereas cassettes might have to be placed in an opening on the top of the machine.

When both hands are safely in the cuffs, the machine may need to be switched on, using a switch which will be near to where your hands are inside the machine. Once you are happy that the rollers are moving you can then unwrap the film. It is worth practising this several times using an exposed film so that you are comfortable with the process and familiar with what is actually inside the film packet. We have all been embarrassed at some stage in our careers to have 'developed' nothing more useful than a piece of black card! Although there is red lighting within the loading part of the processor, you will find it difficult to see the film and have to rely largely on touch to make sure you have the right part of the packet (the film) and feed it into the roller.

Processing the film

The film is moved around the various solutions by rollers or tracks. The film travels through the developer, fixer, and water before it is dried.

Once processed, the film will be collected by the dental nurse from the collection pot.

Digital processing

Digital radiography is now becoming more popular within the dental surgery, but one of its major disadvantages is the financial outlay for the machinery. By using digital technology, the x-ray film is replaced with a flat electronic pad or sensor. The x-rays hit the electronic pad or sensor the same way that they would a traditional film, but rather than manually or automatically developing the film the image is transferred onto a screen. From here, it can be saved or even printed out.

It is essential to monitor the quality of dental radiographs on a regular basis. A simple quality rating tool can be used for this, using a simple numerical system (Table 11.3).

Table 11.3 Simple quality rating tool for dental radiographs

Rating	Quality	Basis
1	Excellent	No errors of patient preparation, exposure, positioning, processing, or film handling
2	Diagnostically acceptable	Some errors of patient preparation, exposure, positioning, processing, or film handling, but which do not detract from the diagnostic utility of the radiograph
3	Unacceptable	Errors of patient preparation, exposure, positioning, processing, or film handling, which render the radiograph diagnostically unacceptable

National Radiological Protection Board/Department of Health 'Guidance notes for dental practitioners on the safe use of x-ray equipment'.

Storing radiographic files and materials

Storing patient x-rays

Mounting

Radiographs can be stored as follows:

- Mounted into acetate sheets by the dental nurse.
- Placed in small envelopes or specially fabricated holders.

The patient's name, date that the x-ray was taken, and, if appropriate, the tooth/teeth should be noted on the films.

Digital radiographs for each patient can be stored on the computer once they have been taken and viewed by the dentist.

Keeping the x-ray on file

Radiographs are stored within the patient's notes, which in turn should be kept in a safe and secure location (see 🛄 The Data Protection Act, p.18).

Storing unexposed film

Unexposed films must be stored as follows:

- Stored away from the X-ray machine, ∴ ensuring they are not accidentally exposed to radiation.
- Kept in a cool, dry environment, such as a stock cupboard.
- New film stock should be placed behind the existing stock. This will ensure that the older films are used before the new films. They should be stored in date order, which will ensure they do not pass the expiry date.

Films that have expired should not be used because this could cause the film to fail and mean that it might have to be retaken.

Film faults: what went wrong?

See Table 11.4 for errors seen on films and suggestions of what might be at fault.

Table 11.4 Description of errors seen on films and suggestions of what might be at fault

Fault	Fault during processing?	Fault taking image?	Action needed
Blank	No film placed into cassette	X-ray set not switched on (more common on new models)	Ensure that all cassettes are checked in the dark room
	Film placed into fixing solution before developer		Ensure solutions are correctly labelled
Partially blank	Straight edge—the film was not fully immersed in the developer	Incorrect angulations of the tube aperture to small. This will show a curve	Ensure the chemicals are at the correct levels before starting
	Curved area—the initial angulation was incorrect or the aperture was too small		
Blurred	N/a	Patient or tube moved	Using the fastest film speed available will ↓ the amount of time that the patient must remain still
Opaque (appears black)	Film overdeveloped	Overexposed	Ensure that the film is placed in the developer for the correct amount of time
	Developer too strong		Ensure the developing solution is made up to the correct dilution
	Developing solution too hot		Check the temperature of the solutions with either a thermometer if manually processing or wait until the light has gone out to indicate the machine is ready if an automatic processor

Transparent (very faint image)	Underdeveloped	Underexposed	Ensure that the film is placed in the developer for the correct amount of time
	Developer too cold		Check the temperature of the solutions with either a thermometer if manually processing or wait until the light has gone out to indicate the machine is ready if an automatic processor
Discoloured	Black spots—film has been contaminated with fixer before being developed	Underexposed	Be careful once the film has been opened to ensure the chemicals do not come in to contact with the film
	White crystals—failed to wash properly after fixing		Ensure that the film is washed properly
	Brown/green areas—incomplete fixing		Ensure the film remains in the fixing solution for the required amount of time
Overlapping teeth	N/a	Angulation of tube incorrect	
Distortion	N/a	Angulation of tube incorrect	

Oral hygiene

Introduction: giving oral hygiene advice

While working as a dental nurse, you might be asked by the dentist to give a patient oral hygiene advice. The type of patient and their needs will determine the type of instructions you will need to give. For example, you might have to give advice to a child who has received a fixed appliance, an adult who has been fitted with a bridge, or an elderly person who has had a new partial denture made.

As a dental nurse, remember that you can only advise patients how to take the best care of their mouth. They might not take kindly to being told what to do.

A dental nurse can give the patient both verbal and written oral hygiene advice and also use models of the teeth and various oral hygiene aids to demonstrate these as well.

Advice on several topics can be given, including the following:
- Brushing the teeth.
- Flossing.
- Interproximal cleaning, using brushes.
- Disclosing tablets.
- Mouthwash.
- Diet analysis.

Please note that the information you give in relation to an individual's oral health needs to be evidence-based. Therefore, *Delivering Better Oral Health*, published by the Department of Health[1] is a useful toolkit to use.

[1] Department of Health & the British Association for the Study of Community Dentistry (2009). *Delivering Better Oral Health*, 2nd edn. London: Department of Health. Available at: ℅ http://www. dh.gov.uk/en/Publicationsandstatistics/Publications/index.htm.

Oral hygiene instruction

Brushing the teeth

Patients can sometimes ask whether a manual or an electric toothbrush is more effective. Unless an effective brushing technique is used, neither type of brush will be of benefit to the patient. Patients should be advised to brush their teeth for a minimum of 2–3 minutes at least twice a day to remove any soft deposits of plaque that have accumulated.

Ideally, the toothbrush should have a small head and medium bristles, ensuring that all the individual surfaces of a tooth can be cleaned. Areas could be missed if the brush is too big and plaque will not be effectively removed if the brush is too soft. All surfaces of each tooth should be cleaned individually. Some advise that the toothbrush should be held at a 45° angle to the tooth; however, the end result following tooth brushing is more important because no technique has been shown to better than another.

It is advised that brushing is supervised until the age of 7. The amount of toothpaste to be used depends on the age of the patient and the need (see Table 12.1).

When using toothpaste containing fluoride, the mouth should not be rinsed after brushing to prolong the beneficial effect of fluoride.

Table 12.1 Amount of toothpaste to be used

Age of patient	Recommended amount of toothpaste	Recommended amount of fluoride in toothpaste
Children up to 3 years old	Small smear	No less than 1000ppm
All children aged 3–6 years	Pea-sized amount	1350–1500ppm
All children and young adults	Pea-sized amount	1350ppm or above
All adult patients	Pea-sized amount	At least 1350ppm

ppm, parts per million.

Flossing

Dental floss can be used to clean the spaces between teeth ('interproximal spaces'). This can take the inexperienced patient a little time to master because it can be fiddly. Patients can also buy dental tape, which is thicker than floss, or super-floss, which is more sponge-like and can be used under bridges. A long length of floss should be dispensed and each end should be wrapped around the middle finger, leaving the index finger and thumb free to manoeuvre the floss between the teeth. The floss should be slid down between the teeth and then down each side of the tooth into the gingival crevice and back out again. This action is repeated with a new section of floss each time. If patients have difficulty using floss, special floss holders can be used. These are small plastic holders to which a piece of floss can be attached.

Interproximal cleaning, using brushes

Interproximal brushes are similar to small bottle brushes and used for cleaning between the teeth. They come in a variety of sizes and the size of the space between the teeth determines the size of the brush to be used. Brushes should be pushed gently between the teeth to remove plaque that has collected there. The brushes should not be forced into the area because this could damage the gingiva.

Disclosing tablets

Disclosing tablets can be used to show a patient the areas/surfaces of the teeth that are being missed during cleaning. After initially brushing the teeth, patients can be encouraged to chew on a disclosing tablet, which will stain any plaque present. The areas that are stained will indicate to the patient the areas they have missed and where more brushing is required.

Mouthwash

A mouthwash can be used daily to support good oral health. Mouthwashes come in a variety of colours and flavours. Some are good for everyday use, whereas others are better for more specialized use. Chlorhexidene-based mouthwashes should not be used on a routine basis because they can stain the teeth. Patients should be advised to use mouthwashes after brushing and follow the manufacturer's instructions.

Diet analysis

A patient's diet can sometimes hold the key to finding out why new cavities are developing. The patient's cleaning technique alone is not always the cause. Patients should be encouraged to complete a diet sheet (Table 12.2), which can be reviewed at their next appointment. Ideally, the diet sheet should cover 2 days at work and 2 days at rest (a weekend or equivalent days off). Once completed, the diet sheet can be analysed to find out what foods and drinks are being consumed and the timeframe between each. Sometimes a patient's diet might seem to be low in sugar but, on careful inspection, hidden sugars are normally forgotten. These can be found in sauces, tinned fruit (in syrup), and certain flavours of crisps. The idea behind diet analysis is to try and help the patient choose alternatives or advise the best time for the patient to eat such foods.

When giving diet advice the dental nurse should consider the patient's general health as well as their oral health. Whilst patients are advised to reduce the amount/frequency of sugar they consume, they should also be advised to maintain a balanced diet. A healthy balanced diet should include food from all the major food groups, preferably of a low fat variety.

Table 12.2 An example of a diet analysis sheet

	3 days during the week	1 weekend day
Date		
Breakfast		
Snacks		
Lunch		
Snacks		
Tea		
Supper		
Bedtime food/drinks		

Antiplaque agents

Both dental caries and periodontal diseases are related to dental plaque. The aims of effective prevention and treatment of these diseases are as follows:

- The patient effectively removing plaque—for periodontal diseases.
- The patient starving the plaque of sugar and other refined carbohydrates by diet modification—for dental caries.
- Strengthening the tooth structure by use of fluoride.

The mainstay of treatment is the removal of plaque and factors that help to retain plaque in the mouth, such as dental calculus and overhanging restorations.

The role of the patient

The most effective way the patient can do this is by use of a toothbrush, toothpaste, and, occasionally, mouthwashes/rinses. The toothbrush is a 'mechanical aid' to plaque removal; that is, it removes plaque through the action of brushing. Various agents can be added to toothpaste or mouthwashes to help plaque removal by chemical means, although these chemicals are, with some exceptions, of limited use in the removal of plaque.

Toothpastes

Ingredients

Toothpastes can contain several ingredients, of which only a few are therapeutic. For example, they might contain the following agents:

- Abrasives—usually very small (microscopic) particles that help polish teeth.
- Detergents—such as sodium lauryl sulphate (SLS), which is a foaming agent.
- Binding agents—such as carboxymethyl cellulose, which stops the separation of the components of the paste.
- Humectants—such as sorbitol, which retains moisture and prevents the paste drying out.
- Flavourings.
- Preservatives—such as benzoates.
- Colouring agents.
- Therapeutic agents:
  - Fluorides.
  - Triclosan.
  - Chlorhexidine.
  - Bicarbonate.
  - Anticalculus agents.
  - Desensitizing agents.

Therapeutic agents

The ideal therapeutic (antiplaque) agent should have the following qualities:

- A broad spectrum of antibacterial activity—that is, the agent should be effective against the wide range of bacteria found in the mouth.
- Substantivity—it should be effective for a long time in the mouth (i.e. stay around and not be washed away too easily).
- Non-toxic.
- Taste pleasant.
- Be compatible with other components of the toothpaste.

Chlorhexidine

The most effective agent in common use is currently chlorhexidine. However, this agent is generally used as a mouthwash (see 📖 Mouthwashes, p.260) rather than a toothpaste, although it is available in a gel (toothpaste-type) form.

Triclosan

Other commonly used agents include triclosan, which is a chlorinated bisphenol and has a broad spectrum of antimicrobial action. Triclosan is often combined in toothpaste with zinc citrate or a copolymer (Gantrez®) to ↑ its efficacy. Triclosan does not prevent the effect of fluoride in toothpaste and, in studies, has been shown to ↓ plaque, gingivitis, and calculus.

Zinc citrate

Might help prevent plaque formation and gingivitis.

Tin

In toothpaste this agent is in the form of 'stannous fluoride', which is antibacterial but stains teeth.

Copper

This agent has some antibacterial properties but also stains teeth.

Mouthwashes

Chlorhexidine mouthwash

The most effective agent; efficacy has been shown in numerous clinical trials.

Properties

Chlorhexidine has the following properties:
- A broad spectrum of activity—effective against bacteria, viruses, and some fungi.
- Low toxicity.
- Substantivity.

Adverse effects

Chlorhexidine stains teeth. If the agent is used in toothpaste, this effect is more pronounced and it might cause the formation of calculus.

The agent might also cause taste disturbance and, occasionally, redness and soreness of the oral soft tissues.

Uses

- Chlorhexidine is very effective at preventing plaque, but it does not remove it.
- It might be inactivated by foaming agents (SLS) in toothpastes.
- It can be combined with fluoride in mouthwashes, but this is not so easy in toothpastes because of the chemistry.
- Chlorhexidine has been used in chewing gum, when less staining was noted.
- It might also help control aphthous ulceration.
- Chlorhexidine is also available in a spray for certain patients.

Indications

Chlorhexidine should be used in the following circumstances:
- For patients who cannot carry out mechanical plaque control.
- Immediately before and in the weeks following oral surgery.
- To ↓ the risk of oral candidiasis (thrush).
- In immunocompromised patients.
- Patients at very high risk of caries.
- Patients with recurrent aphthous ulceration.

Fluoride mouthwashes

- Can be only be recommended by a dentist following an assessment of the patient.
- Are for daily or weekly use depending on the circumstances.
- Are for patients aged 8 years and above.
- They are used as an adjunct to brushing with a toothpaste containing fluoride.

Other mouthwashes

Although chlorhexidine is the most effective antiplaque agent, several other mouthwashes that have been tested for their antiplaque effect are available.

Sanguinarine

- Made from an alcoholic extract of the blood-root plant.
- Retained in plaque for a few hours.
- Sanguinarine might ↓ or inhibit plaque formation but not gingivitis.
- Seems more effective as a mouthwash than a toothpaste.

Cetylpyridinium chloride

- Quaternary ammonium compound.
- Little proven effectiveness.
- Poor substantivity.

Povidine iodine

- Little evidence for its effectiveness as a mouthwash, but useful as an irrigator in certain patients, such as those with HIV or ANUG.
- ↓ the discomfort of ulceration.
- Not to be used during pregnancy or in patients with thyroid problems.

Hexetidine

- Low antiplaque activity.
- Might cause ulceration if the agent is in >1% solution.

Essential oils

- Essential oils such as thymol, menthol, and eucalyptol have been used in mouth rinses for >100 years.
- These have been shown to be antibacterial in laboratory tests.
- The essential oils of clove, cinnamon, and thyme have significant effects against >20 types of bacteria.

Restorative dentistry

Introduction: restorative dentistry

Restorative dentistry, as the name implies, is concerned with the preservation of sound tooth tissue and the removal and replacement of diseased tooth tissue with a variety of suitable materials using a multitude of techniques.

Why would a tooth need to be restored?

- Dental caries.
- Loss of tooth surface from abrasion, attrition, or erosion.
- The tooth has broken as a result of trauma.

Aims of restorative treatment

- Remove diseased tissue.
- Prevent further destruction of remaining tooth structure.
- Restore the function of the tooth.
- Restore the appearance of the tooth.

There are many different types of dental materials that can be used to restore a tooth. The types of restorative materials used will depend on the extent of the damage to the tooth and its location within the oral cavity.

This chapter contains descriptions of tooth restoration procedures. Further information regarding the individual materials can be found in Chapter 17.

Cavity preparation

The removal of diseased tissue, as a first step in restoring teeth affected by caries, results in cavities of varying shapes and sizes. These cavities must be modified according to the following:

- The properties of the restorative material to be used.
- The tooth affected.
- The surface of the tooth affected.
- Whether the cavity involves >1 surface.

Choosing a restorative material

In general, cavities in posterior teeth are restored with amalgam or gold because strength, rather than appearance, is the main concern. However, in anterior teeth, appearance is the main factor. Materials that are the same colour as the tooth are used, such as composite or glass ionomer (or both in combination).

Classification of cavities

There are several classifications of cavities in use, the oldest of which is Black's classification, which is based on the location of a cavity on a tooth. In this classification there are 5 classes (I–V; Table 13.1). Other classifications use descriptive terms, such as occlusal and labial cavities.

Cavity design

Some dental materials, such as amalgam, cannot bond directly to the surface of the tooth and must be retained mechanically in the cavity. This can be achieved by cutting cavities with specific design features, e.g. making the inside of the cavity bigger than its opening so that, when the cavity is filled with amalgam and allowed to set, it will not fall out. Such a cavity feature is called an 'undercut'.

Table 13.1 Black's classifications

Class I	Caries affecting pits and fissures of posterior (premolar/molar) teeth
Class II	Caries affecting 2 of the tooth surfaces, the mesial or distal and the occlusal surface of a posterior tooth
Class III	Caries affecting the mesial or distal surfaces of anterior (incisor/canine) teeth
Class IV	Caries affecting the mesial or distal surfaces of anterior teeth and extending to the incisal edge
Class V	Caries affecting the cervical margins (area at the neck of the tooth)

Amalgam restorations

Amalgam is one of the oldest and most commonly used materials for restoring posterior teeth. It is made from an alloy powder that is mixed with liquid mercury. Amalgam initially sets within a few minutes but it does not set completely until a few hours later (see 📖 Amalgam, p.354).

Dental caries might be extensive and affect >1 surface of the tooth. The cavity is not surrounded by cavity walls so amalgam can not be packed easily without spilling. In those cases, amalgam must be contained while it is being packed into the cavity by use of a 'matrix band' held in place with a 'matrix band retainer' and 'wedges'.

Stages during the procedure

- Administer a local anaesthetic to the patient.
- Place a rubber dam.
- Remove caries by use of a contra-angle hand piece and round steel latch-grip bur.
- Prepare the cavity using a fast handpiece and diamond- or tungsten carbide-tipped friction-grip bur.
- Insert a suitable cavity liner to protect the pulp from thermal shock and chemical irritation.
- If required, place a matrix band and retainer onto the tooth.
- Insert the amalgam using the amalgam carrier and pack it into the cavity with an amalgam plugger.
- Trim any excess amalgam and shape it using a carver.
- Use a straight probe and dental floss to remove excess material.
- Check the occlusion using articulating paper—remove any high spots and smooth the surface by use of a burnisher.

Role of the dental nurse

- Collect the patient notes and identify the planned procedure.
- Prepare the clinical environment.
- Prepare the relevant instruments, materials, and equipment needed for the procedure, including PPE for the dental team and patient.
- Select and prepare the local anaesthetic and pass it to the dentist.
- Aspirate and retract the soft tissues to maintain a clear field of vision and remove debris while the cavity is being prepared.
- Prepare the appropriate lining material and pass it to the dentist with an applicator.
- Mix the amalgam in the amalgamator and place it into a dappen pot. Load the amalgam into an amalgam carrier and pass it to the dentist. Repeat until the cavity is filled.
- Pass the amalgam plugger and carver when required.
- Place the articulating paper into the Miller forceps and pass these to the dentist to check the occlusion.
- Monitor and reassure the patient throughout the procedure.
- Provide aftercare instruction to the patient.

Instruments and materials

- Mirror, straight probe, tweezers, amalgam plugger, carver, burnisher, Miller forceps, contra-angle and fast handpieces, and a selection of burs.
- Rubber dam kit and aspirator tip/saliva ejector.
- Local anaesthetic cartridge, syringe, and needle.
- Dappen pot and amalgam carrier, articulating paper, matrix band and retainer, and lining applicator.
- Amalgam and lining material.

Amalgam is produced by mixing an alloy powder and mercury. The mercury liquid is toxic. Precautions must be taken to minimize exposure to mercury vapour (see 🔲 Mercury poisoning, p.356).

This applies not only during placement of new restorations, but also during removal of old restorations.

Aftercare instructions

At the end of the procedure, the dental nurse should offer the patient a mouthwash and wipe and remove the patient's PPE. Patients should be advised that amalgam restorations take 24 hours to set hard and they should avoid biting down too heavily because this might cause the restoration to fracture. Also, if a local anaesthetic has been given, the area will be numb for a couple of hours so they should avoid hot food or drinks to prevent burning the soft tissues of the mouth or biting their lip/tongue.

Composite restorations

Composite material: pros and cons

Composites are the same colour as teeth and ideal for restoring cavities where appearance is important, such as for anterior teeth. Composite materials come in a variety of shades, enabling the dentist to pick one that matches the shade of the tooth being treated. A guide to composite shades can be used to compare the composite with the patient's own teeth and select the appropriate shade.

Unlike amalgam, composites can be made to bond directly to the enamel by use of the acid-etch technique or a bonding agent, which aids bonding to the dentine.

For setting, composites can be light, chemical, or dual cured.

Stages during the procedure

- Administer a local anaesthetic, place rubber dam and remove caries and prepare the cavity as done when placing an amalgam restoration (see 🕮 Amalgam restorations, p.266).
- Prepare the cavity using a fast handpiece and diamond- or tungsten carbide-tipped friction-grip bur.
- Insert a suitable cavity liner to protect the pulp from chemical irritation.
- Etchant is used to etch the enamel—this is left for the recommended amount of time and then washed off.
- If required, use a bonding agent—this is applied to the tooth and cured (by light or chemical means).
- Note the shade of the tooth using a shade guide and select the appropriate composite.
- Place the composite in small increments and set it using light or chemical curing.
- A clear matrix strip might be needed to complete the restoration.
- Check the occlusion using articulating paper and adjust as necessary.
- If happy with the restoration, the dentist will finish and polish the restoration with finishing/polishing strips or discs.

Role of the dental nurse

- Collect the patient notes and identify the planned procedure.
- Prepare the clinical environment.
- Prepare the relevant instruments, materials, and equipment needed for the procedure, including PPE for the dental team and patient (the patient will require special shaded glasses to protect their eyes from the light cure. Orange-coloured glass is used to shield the light to protect the dental team while using curing light).
- Select and prepare the local anaesthetic and it pass to the dentist.
- Aspirate and retract the soft tissues to maintain a clear field of vision and remove debris while the cavity is being prepared.
- Prepare and hand the dentist the etchant—aspirate while the etchant is rinsed off.
- Place the bond into a dappen pot and hand this to the dentist with an applicator—provide the curing light and hold the orange shield.

- Assist the dentist in taking the shade of the tooth and select the appropriate shade of composite.
- Prepare the composite and hand it to the dentist with a flat plastic instrument—pass more of the material until the restoration is complete.
- If a dual- or light-cured composite is used, pass the light to the dentist as required.
- Place articulating paper into the Miller forceps and pass these to the dentist to check the occlusion.
- The dental nurse might need to aspirate while the restoration is adjusted and finished.
- Monitor and reassure the patient throughout the procedure.
- Provide aftercare instructions to the patient.

Instruments and materials required

- Mirror, straight probe, tweezers, flat plastic Miller forceps, contra-angle and fast handpieces, a selection of burs, lining applicator, mandrel, and polishing/finishing discs or strips.
- Rubber dam kit and aspirator tip/saliva ejector.
- Local anaesthetic cartridge, syringe, and needle.
- Light cure and orange shield.
- Dappen pots, applicator brushes, articulating paper, clear matrix strip, composite, etchant, bonding agent, and lining material.

❶ The light used to set the composite can damage the eyes of the patient, dentist, and nurse. The patient's eyes must be protected by use of sunglasses and those of the dentist and nurse by shielding the light with orange-coloured light filters.

❶ The tip of the curing light can come into contact with the tooth and must be covered with fresh clingfilm to avoid cross-infection.

❶ The matrix band used during placement of composite restorations must allow the light rays from the machine to reach the material. These matrix bands must be transparent.

Aftercare instructions

These are similar to those given after placing an amalgam restoration (see Amalgam restoration, p.266).

Glass ionomer restorations

Glass ionomer materials are 'tooth'-coloured and can be placed where appearance is important. The materials come in different shades so can be matched to the tooth being treated. However, the material is inferior to composite in terms of appearance and surface finish.

Glass ionomer cement can bond to dentine, making it suitable for cavities where retention can be difficult to obtain. A dentine conditioner should be used before placement to ensure the dentine surface is free from any debris that could stop the material sticking to the tooth effectively.

Glass ionomer materials can be chemically or light cured.

Moisture can affect the setting of the material so moisture control is important during placement (see 📖 Glass ionomer cement, p.358).

Stages during the procedure

- Administer a local anaesthetic, place rubber dam, and remove caries as for amalgam and composite (see 📖 Amalgam restorations, p.266).
- If required, place an appropriate lining material.
- Place conditioner onto the dentine.
- Select the appropriate shade of material using a shade guide.
- Place the glass ionomer material and light cure, if necessary.
- Place a clear matrix band over the restoration and set it using light or chemical curing.
- Apply the varnish supplied with the kit or use a thin layer of composite to protect the set restoration.

Role of the dental nurse

- Collect the patient notes and identify the planned procedure.
- Prepare the clinical environment.
- Prepare the relevant instruments, materials, and equipment needed for the procedure, including PPE for the dental team and patient.
- Select and prepare the local anaesthetic and pass it to the dentist.
- Aspirate and retract the soft tissues to maintain a clear field of vision and remove debris while the cavity is being prepared.
- Prepare the lining material, if required, and pass it to the dentist with the lining applicator.
- Place conditioner into a dappen pot and hand to the dentist with an applicator—aspirate while the conditioner is rinsed and dried.
- Prepare the required amount of glass ionomer material and pass it to the dentist with a flat plastic instrument—hand the dentist a clear matrix strip, if required.
- Check the time if chemical curing is used or pass the light cure to the dentist to set the material.
- Pass the varnish to the dentist in a dappen pot, with an applicator brush.

Instruments and materials required

- Mirror, straight probe, tweezers, flat plastic Miller forceps, contra-angle and fast handpieces, a selection of burs, and lining applicator.
- Rubber dam kit and aspirator tip/saliva ejector.
- Local anaesthetic cartridge, syringe, and needle.
- Light cure and orange shield.
- Dappen pots, applicator brushes, articulating paper, clear matrix strip, composite, tooth conditioner, varnish or composite, and lining material.

Aftercare instructions

These are similar to those given for after placing amalgam restorations (see 📖 Amalgam restorations, p.266).

❶ The setting reaction of glass ionomer cement takes 24 hours to complete, during which time it is vulnerable to contamination with saliva or water. Hence, the need for protection.

❶ Covering the restoration with petroleum jelly does not give adequate protection.

Acid-etch technique

Composites can be bonded to enamel by use of this technique.

Etchants contain a weak acid, such as phosphoric acid, which is applied directly to the enamel. The acid dissolves the surface, forming tiny holes. The etchant is washed off and composite is placed on top—the composite flows into the tiny holes, which help it adhere to the enamel surface.

Etchant can cause damage to the soft tissues. These must be adequately protected during the procedure, by good aspiration or cotton-wool rolls, to prevent damage occurring (see ◻ Etchants, p.361).

Stages of the procedure
- Remove all caries.
- Wash and dry the enamel surface.
- Apply the etchant to the tooth using an applicator brush.
- Leave the etchant on the tooth for the time recommended by the manufacturer's instructions.
- The 3-in-1 (see Chapter 8) is then used to rinse the etchant off the tooth.

Role of the dental nurse
- Place the etchant into a dappen pot and hand it to the dentist, with an applicator brush.
- Alert the dentist when the etchant has been on the tooth for the correct amount of time.
- Aspirate while the etchant is rinsed off.

- The etchant is coloured to help the dentist apply it only to the area of enamel to be etched.
- The duration of etching is crucial—the nurse must keep time carefully.

Instruments and materials required
- Mirror, straight probe, tweezers, and rubber dam kit.
- Local anaesthetic cartridge, syringe, and needle.
- Dappen pots, applicator brushes, cotton-wool rolls, etchant material, and aspirator tips/saliva ejector.

Temporary restorations

In some cases (e.g. emergency treatment, preparation of an inlay or veneer, or root-canal treatment), a permanent restoration cannot be placed directly into a tooth. Temporary restorations are carried out to prevent further damage to the tooth surfaces until a permanent restoration can be placed.

Materials

Temporary materials are fairly strong but too soft or soluble to be used as permanent restoration material. The following materials can be used for temporary restorations:

- Zinc oxide and eugenol (ZOE) cement.
- Polycarboxylate cement.
- Zinc phosphate cement.
- Glass ionomer cement (see 🕮 Glass ionomer cement, p.358).

Properties

These materials usually come in the form of a powder and liquid which are mixed together to the desired consistency. There are some ready-mixed forms available but these might prove to be more costly than self-mix versions.

When a temporary material is used, the dentist will simply place the material into the cavity, pack it into place with a plugger, and trim off any excess. The patient is asked to bite down on the material while it is still soft so it moulds to the correct height.

❶ The patient should be warned that the material is only a temporary measure and they should return to the surgery to have it replaced if it falls out or fractures. They should also be told that some materials (e.g. ZOE) might also discolour if coffee, red wines, and some highly coloured foods (e.g. curries) are consumed.

Inlays: first visit

For restorations with amalgam, composite, and glass ionomer cement, the material is placed in the cavity and made to harden *in situ*. By contrast, 'inlays' are restorations that are constructed in a laboratory by a dental technician.

When preparing the cavity, the walls must be made parallel to enable the inlay to be fitted and cemented into place.

Inlays can be constructed out of a metal material, such as gold (for strength), or in different shades of porcelain (for appearance). Inlays are used for teeth that have lost cusps or if amalgam is not strong enough to restore the tooth.

Making inlays occurs in several stages and will require a minimum of 2 visits by the patient.

Stages of the procedure

- Administer a local anaesthetic, place rubber dam, and remove caries and prepare cavity as done during placement of an amalgam restoration (see ☐ Amalgam restorations, p.266).
- Take an impression of the opposing arch using alginate and a wax squash bite to record the occlusion—use an elastomer or silicone impression material to take an impression of the prepared cavity.
- Take a record of the occlusion modelling wax.
- If a porcelain inlay is to be made, take a shade using a shade guide.
- Place a temporary material into the cavity.
- Disinfect the impression materials and place them into a bag.
- A detailed prescription accompanies the impression to be sent to the laboratory for the construction of the inlay—attach it to the bag.
- Give the patient aftercare instructions and make a further appointment for fitting the inlay.

Role of the dental nurse

- Collect the patient notes and identify the planned procedure.
- Prepare the clinical environment.
- Prepare the relevant instruments, materials, and equipment needed for the procedure, including PPE for the dental team and patient.
- Select and prepare the local anaesthetic and pass it to the dentist.
- Aspirate and retract the soft tissues to maintain a clear field of vision and remove debris while the cavity is being prepared.
- Select appropriate impression trays, apply tray adhesive, and attach the handle.
- Mix the required amount of alginate impression material, load it into a tray, and pass it to the dentist.
- Prepare the elastomer material and load it into an impression tray.
- Monitor and reassure the patient while the impression material is in their mouth.
- Take modelling wax and roll into an arch shape and hand it to the dentist.

- Disinfect the impressions and wax bite and place them into a plastic bag.
- Prepare the temporary restoration material and pass it to the dentist with a flat plastic.
- Give the patient aftercare instructions.
- Ensure the laboratory card is completed and arrange a further appointment for the patient.

Instruments and materials required

- Mirror, straight probe, tweezers, contra-angle and fast handpieces, and a selection of burs.
- Impression trays, tray handles, tray adhesive, alginate and elastomer/silicone materials, mixing spatulas, mixing bowl, water measuring cup, mixing pad, temporary restoration material, modelling wax, and a heat source.
- Shade guide, laboratory bag, and card.

Aftercare instructions

These are similar to those given after placing an amalgam restoration (see ▢ Amalgam restorations, p.266).

❶ Close liaison with the laboratory is required so that the patient's next appointment coincides with the delivery of the completed inlay.

The patient must be made aware that they should return to have the temporary restoration replaced if it falls out, because it protects the underlying tooth surfaces until the inlay is fitted.

Inlays: second visit

Stages of the procedure

- Administer a local anaesthetic to the patient.
- Place a rubber dam—this might not be used sometimes.
- Remove the temporary restoration material.
- Try the permanent inlay in the cavity to check it fits—margins, bite (occlusion), and colour (if porcelain).
- Adjust the inlay, if necessary, and then repolish it.
- Cement the inlay into the cavity.
- Remove excess cement.
- Recheck the bite using articulating paper.
- Give the patient aftercare instructions.

Role of the dental nurse

- Collect the patient notes and identify the planned procedure.
- Prepare the clinical environment.
- Prepare the relevant instruments, materials, and equipment needed for the procedure, including PPE for the dental team and patient—ensure the inlay is also prepared.
- Aspirate and retract the soft tissues to maintain a clear field of vision and remove debris while the temporary is removed.
- Prepare the appropriate cement and pass it to the dentist with a flat plastic.
- Aspirate while excess cement is removed.
- Place the articulating paper into the Miller forceps and pass these to the dentist to check the occlusion.
- Provide the patient with aftercare instructions.

❶ The dental nurse should ensure that the inlay has returned from the laboratory before the patient's appointment, so that if it has not, the patient's appointment can be rearranged. The patient will not be happy if they come for their appointment and it has to be cancelled because the inlay isn't there.

Instruments and materials required

- Mirror, straight probe, tweezers, contra-angle and fast handpieces, and a selection of burs.
- Inlay, permanent cement, mixing pad, spatula, aspirator tip/saliva ejector, articulating paper, and Miller forceps.

Aftercare instructions

These are similar to those given after placing an amalgam restoration (see 📖 Amalgam restorations, p.266).

Veneers: first visit

A veneer is similar to a false nail; that is, it is a thin layer of porcelain (only 0.5mm thick) that covers the visible labial or buccal (front) surface of a tooth. It is a procedure used to gain good aesthetics (appearance). For example, a veneer can be used to correct teeth that are discoloured, out of alignment, rotated, or have large gaps between them.

Veneers are normally fitted on the upper and lower incisal and canine teeth, because they are not strong enough to withstand the biting action of the molars and premolars, and also because they can't be easily seen and aren't an aesthetic issue. Porcelain can be made in many shades so it can be closely matched to the patient's own adjacent teeth. Veneers are bonded to acid-etched enamel by use of composite cement. Because the veneers are made in a laboratory, 2 patient visits are needed.

Stages of the procedure

- Administer a local anaesthetic to the patient.
- Record the shade.
- Take an impression of the tooth with silicone putty to make a temporary veneer later.
- Place a rubber dam—this may not be used sometimes.
- Prepare the tooth using a fast handpiece and diamond- or tungsten carbide-tipped friction-grip bur.
- Use elastomer or silicone impression materials to take an impression of the prepared tooth.
- Make a temporary veneer with composite using the putty impression taken previously.
- Bond the temporary veneer using the acid-etch technique but taking care only to etch small spots of the prepared enamel surface ('spot etching').
- Check the fit of the temporary veneer and cement it into place.
- Give the patient aftercare instructions.
- Disinfect the impression materials and placed them into a bag.
- Write a detailed prescription to accompany the impression for the construction of the veneer and attach it to the bag.

Role of the dental nurse

- Collect the patient notes and identify the planned procedure.
- Prepare the clinical environment.
- Prepare the relevant instruments, materials, and equipment needed for the procedure, including PPE for the dental team and patient.
- Select and prepare the local anaesthetic and pass it to the dentist.
- Assist the dentist in taking the shade.
- Select appropriate impression trays, apply tray adhesive, and attach the handle.
- Mix the required amount of elastomer/silicone impression material, load it into the tray, and pass it to the dentist.
- Aspirate and retract the soft tissues to maintain a clear field of vision and remove debris while the tooth is prepared.

- Select appropriate impression trays, apply tray adhesive, and attach the handle. Then, prepare the elastomer material and load in to an impression tray.
- Monitor and reassure the patient while the impression material is in their mouth.
- Disinfect the impressions and place them into a plastic bag.
- Prepare the etchant and pass it to the dentist in a dappen pot, with an applicator.
- Pass the composite material, load into impression, and pass to the dentist.
- Give the patient aftercare instructions.
- Ensure the laboratory card is completed and arrange a further appointment for the patient.

Instruments and materials required

- Mirror, straight probe, tweezers, contra-angle and fast handpieces, and a selection of burs.
- Impression trays, tray handles, tray adhesive, elastomer/silicone materials, composite, acid etch, dappen pot, and applicator brush.
- Shade guide, laboratory bag, and card.

Aftercare instructions

These are similar to those given after placing an amalgam restoration (see ▢ Amalgam restorations, p.266).

Veneers: second visit

Stages of the procedure

- Administer local analgesia.
- Remove the temporary veneer and any temporary cement and then wash and dry the tooth.
- Try the permanent veneer and adjust, if necessary.
- Acid etch the tooth surface and then wash and dry it.
- Cement the veneer into place.
- Check the final fit.
- Give the patient aftercare instructions.

Role of the dental nurse

- Collect the patient notes and identify the planned procedure.
- Prepare the clinical environment.
- Prepare the relevant instruments, materials, and equipment needed for the procedure, including PPE for the dental team and patient—ensure the veneer is also prepared.
- Aspirate and retract the soft tissues to maintain a clear field of vision and remove debris while the temporary is removed and the tooth is cleaned and dried.
- Prepare the appropriate cement and pass it to the dentist with a flat plastic.
- Allow time for the cement to set or pass the curing light.
- Aspirate while excess cement is removed.
- Provide the patient with aftercare instructions.

❶ Veneers can be inhaled or swallowed by the patient. The nurse must be careful and vigilant.

Veneers are fragile and must be handled with care. They are bonded to enamel with light-cured composite to give adequate working time. However, the translucency of the veneer might not be enough to let enough light to pass through, leading to poor setting of the composite. Dual-cure composites, which set by light activation and chemical reaction, are better.

Instruments and materials required

- Mirror, straight probe, tweezers, contra-angle and fast handpieces, and a selection of burs.
- Inlay, permanent cement, mixing pad, spatula, aspirator tip/saliva ejector, articulating paper, and Miller forceps.

Aftercare instructions

These are similar to those given after placing an amalgam restoration (see ⎙ Amalgam restorations, p.266). In addition, patients should be told that veneers are fragile and they should not bite down heavily on foods such as apples, carrots, and any other hard foods or the veneer could fracture.

Crowns

Crowns are called caps by patients. They cover all surfaces of the crown of a tooth. They can be made of gold or porcelain, or a combination of both:
- Gold crowns—posterior teeth.
- Porcelain crowns—anterior teeth.
- Porcelain bonded to metal crowns—both anterior and posterior teeth.

The teeth need preparation to accommodate crowns.

First visit
- Diagnosis and treatment planning.
- Local analgesia.
- Record the shade if a porcelain or metal–ceramic crown is used.
- Take an impression of the tooth with silicone putty to make a temporary crown later.
- Tooth preparation.
- Take an impression.
- Record the bite or occlusion.
- Fabrication of a temporary crown using the silicone putty impression taken earlier.
- Cementation of a temporary crown.
- Checking and finishing.
- Instruct the patient on aftercare before discharging them.
- Write a detailed prescription (e.g. the design and shade of metal–ceramic crown) to accompany the impressions and occlusal record to be sent to the laboratory.

❶ The impression must be disinfected before sending to the laboratory.

Second visit
- Local analgesia.
- Remove the temporary crown and cement and then wash and dry.
- Try the permanent crown—check the fit, margins, occlusion, and shade and adjust, if necessary.
- Re-polish the crown.
- Cement the crown.
- Checking and finishing.
- Instruct the patient on aftercare before discharging them.

❶ Although crowns, in general, are larger than veneers, they can still be inhaled or swallowed by the patient. The nurse must be careful and vigilant.

Instruments and materials required
- Mirror, straight probe, tweezers, contra-angle and fast handpieces, and a selection of burs.
- Impression trays, tray handles, tray adhesive, alginate and elastomer/silicone materials, mixing spatulas, mixing bowl, water measuring cup, mixing pad, temporary restoration material, modelling wax, gingival retraction cord, and a heat source.
- Shade guide, laboratory bag, and card.

Bridges

Bridges are used to replace missing teeth. They serve the same function as a partial denture, except that bridges are permanently fixed to teeth.

If a tooth is missing, the 2 teeth on either side can be used to retain the bridge, replacing the missing tooth. The part of the bridge replacing the missing tooth is called the 'pontic' and the parts fixed to the 2 teeth on either side (the 'abutment' teeth) are called 'retainers'. In general, crowns are used as retainers. Provision of a bridge entails preparation of teeth on either side of the gap for crowns to be used as retainers.

Bridge designs

If both teeth on either side of the gap are used for retention, then the bridge has a 'fixed–fixed' design. If the pontic is attached to 1 of the retainers by a joint that permits some movement, then the bridge has a 'fixed–movable' design. A single pontic with 2 retainers will make up a 3-unit bridge. Dentists are conscious of the need to preserve teeth and, if other factors (e.g. occlusion, quality of the abutment teeth, and periodontal health) permit, only 1 abutment tooth can be used to retain the bridge. Such a bridge is called a 'cantilever bridge'.

Resin-retained bridge

This is an innovation that combines the effectiveness of the acid-etch technique with the need to preserve as much tooth tissue as possible. In this design, conventional crowns are not used as bridge retainers. Instead, teeth are prepared minimally, involving only the enamel (hence the alternative term 'minimum-preparation bridge'), and the retainers bonded to the prepared abutment teeth by use of the acid-etch technique. In general, such bridges are limited to 3 units. Nevertheless, they can be of fixed–fixed, fixed–movable, or a 2-unit cantilever design.

First visit

- Diagnosis and treatment planning.
- Impressions of both arches.
- Recording the occlusion.
- Recording the shade of teeth.
- Writing a detailed prescription to accompany the impressions and the occlusal record to be sent to the laboratory.

❶ The impressions must be disinfected before sending to the laboratory.

Laboratory stage

- Cast impressions.
- Mount the casts on a suitable articulator using the occlusal record taken.
- Design the bridge.

Second visit

- Local analgesia.
- Taking a putty impression of abutment teeth.
- Preparation of abutment teeth.
- Taking an impression.
- Recording the occlusion.
- Fabrication of a temporary bridge using the putty impression taken previously.
- Checking and cementing the temporary bridge using temporary cement.
- Instructing the patient on aftercare before discharging them.
- Writing a detailed prescription (e.g. design of the bridge, whether retainers are to be used, and shade) to accompany the impressions and occlusal record to be sent to the laboratory.

Laboratory stage

- Casting of impressions.
- Mounting of casts on an articulator using the occlusal records.
- Waxing of the bridge, according to the design prescribed.
- Casting the metal framework.
- Adding porcelain where appropriate and firing.
- Checking and finishing.

Third visit

- Removing the temporary bridge.
- Cleaning, washing, and drying abutment teeth.
- Trying the bridge—checking the fit, margins, occlusion, and shade.
- Adjusting the bridge, if necessary, and re-polishing.
- Cementing the bridge and checking again.
- Instructing the patient on aftercare and cleaning instructions before discharging them.

Instruments and materials required

- Mirror, straight probe, tweezers, contra-angle and fast handpieces, and a selection of burs.
- Bridge, permanent cement, mixing pad, spatula, aspirator tip/saliva ejector, articulating paper, and Miller forceps.

Temporary crowns and bridges

(Also see 📖 Temporary materials, p.362.)

Provision of crowns and bridges for teeth involves several stages spread over several patient visits. For example, to provide a full veneer crown, the tooth must be cut or prepared first to a specific design and an impression taken of the cut tooth, which is sent to a laboratory for fabrication of the crown (a process that can take several days). In the meantime, the cut tooth cannot be left unprotected, so a temporary crown is made and cemented into place until the permanent crown is available for cementation.

Temporary crowns

These can be custom-made by taking an impression of the tooth before cutting it. This impression, usually taken with silicone putty, can be used to make a provisional crown similar in shape and size to the original tooth. After the preparation of the tooth is complete, the silicone putty impression is filled with a suitable temporary crown material and accurately reseated. Once the material has partially set, the impression is removed and the material allowed to set completely. Then the provisional crown is prised free from the putty and any excess removed. The crown is then tried and checked for fit, margins, and occlusion. Adjustments are made, if necessary. Once the impression for the permanent crown is taken successfully, the temporary crown is cemented with temporary cement.

Temporary crowns can also be made using ready-made hollow-shell crowns or crown forms. They must be lined on the inside with temporary crown material, seated on the prepared tooth to mould the material to shape, and allowed to set. Then it is removed, excess material removed, checked again, and adjusted, if necessary, before temporary cementation.

Temporary bridges

These are used to protect prepared abutment teeth, in addition to maintaining the space left by the missing teeth until the bridge is made. The procedure is similar to making a temporary crown, except that the missing teeth also must be incorporated into the structure. For this reason, the putty impression is taken of the cast, with the missing teeth replaced by suitable denture teeth. Once the abutment teeth have been prepared, the putty impression is lined with temporary bridge material, including the spaces occupied by denture teeth, and carefully reseated. Once the material has partially set, the impression is removed, allowed to set completely, and the temporary bridge prised free. Any excess material is removed. The temporary bridge is then tried for fit, margins, and occlusion and adjusted, if necessary, polished, and cemented with temporary cement into place.

Instruments and materials required

- Mirror, straight probe, tweezers, contra-angle and fast handpieces, and a selection of burs.
- Temporary cement, temporary bridge material, impression material and trays, mixing pad, spatula, aspirator tip/saliva ejector, articulating paper, and Miller forceps.

Full dentures

These are removable appliances used to replace all the missing teeth in a jaw. They are made of acrylic alone or in combination with cobalt chromium alloy (see 📖 Immediate dentures, p.290, for cases where remaining teeth are present).

First visit

- Diagnosis and treatment planning.
- Taking impressions using stock trays and alginate impression material (or other suitable material).
- Writing a detailed prescription to accompany the impressions to be sent to the laboratory.

❶ The impression must be disinfected before sending to the laboratory.

Instruments and materials required
- Mirror, straight probe, tweezers.
- Impression material, mixing bowl, spatula, selection of trays, tray handles, water, aspirator tip/saliva ejector.

Laboratory stage
- Casting impressions.
- Making special trays.

Second visit

- Taking master impressions using the special trays and silicone impression material.
- Recording jaw relationships by use of a facebow (a metal caliper-like device).
- Writing a detailed prescription to accompany the impressions and occlusal record to be sent to the laboratory.

❶ The impression must be disinfected before sending to the laboratory.

Instruments and materials required
- Mirror, straight probe, tweezers, contra-angle, straight and fast handpieces, and a selection of burs (for adjusting trays).
- Facebow with attachments.
- Impression material, mixing pad, spatula, modelling wax, aspirator tip/ saliva ejector.

Laboratory stage
- Casting master impressions.
- Mounting the casts in an articulator using the occlusal records.
- Making wax rims.

Third visit

- Measuring the lower face height at rest and freeway space by use of a Willis bite gauge or pair of dividers.
- Inserting wax rims and adjusting them to get the correct contour, lower face height with bite rims in occlusion.
- Marking the midline, canine lines, and lip lines.
- Sealing the wax rims together and removing them from the patient's mouth.
- Selecting the mould and shade of the teeth.
- Writing a detailed prescription to accompany the impressions and occlusal record to be sent to the laboratory.

Instruments and materials required
- Mirror, straight probe, tweezers.
- Modeling wax, Willis bite gauge or a pair of dividers, Fox's occlusal plane guide, wax knife, LeCron carver, Heat source, shade guide.
- Aspirator tip/saliva ejector, articulating paper, and Miller forceps.

Laboratory stage
- Setting the teeth.

Fourth visit

- Trying the trial dentures.
- Checking the appearance, occlusion, lower face height, and freeway space.
- Obtaining consent to proceed from the patient.
- Writing a detailed prescription to accompany the trial dentures to be sent to the laboratory.

Instruments and materials required
- Mirror, straight probe, tweezers, contra-angle, straight and fast handpieces, and a selection of burs.
- Wax knife, Lecron carver, modeling wax, heat source, shade guide.
- Aspirator tip/saliva ejector, articulating paper, and Miller forceps.

Fifth visit

- Fitting the dentures.
- Checking the appearance, occlusion, and patient's speech and adjusting, if required.
- Instructing the patient on aftercare before discharging them.

Instruments and materials required
- Mirror, straight probe, tweezers, contra-angle and straight handpieces, and a selection of burs.
- Pressure indicator paste.
- Aspirator tip/saliva ejector, articulating paper, and Miller forceps.

Partial dentures

These are removable appliances that replace a few missing teeth, similar to bridges and full dentures. They can be made of acrylic or cobalt chromium alloy. The acrylic partial dentures are cheaper; ∴ more of these are made.

First visit
- Diagnosis and treatment planning.
- Periodontal treatment.
- Extracting teeth with poor prognosis and restoring other teeth.

Second visit
- Taking impressions using stock trays and alginate impression material.
- Recording jaw relationships with occlusal records and a facebow.
- Writing a detailed prescription to accompany the impressions to be sent to the laboratory.

❶ The impression must be disinfected before sending to the laboratory.

Instruments and materials required
- Mirror, straight probe, tweezers.
- Impression material, mixing bowl, spatula, selection of trays, tray handles, water, aspirator tip/saliva ejector.

Laboratory stage
- Casting 1° impressions.
- Making special trays.
- Mounting casts on an articulator using the occlusal records and a facebow.
- Designing the dentures.

Third visit
- Preparing teeth selected for denture support and retention.
- Taking master impressions using the special trays and silicone impression material.
- Recording jaw relationships with a facebow.
- Writing a detailed prescription (e.g. design of dentures, teeth to be clasped, and occlusal rests) to accompany the impressions and occlusal record to be sent to the laboratory.

❶ The impression must be disinfected before sending to the laboratory.

Instruments and materials required
- Mirror, straight probe, tweezers, contra-angle, straight and fast handpieces, and a selection of burs (for adjusting trays).
- Facebow with attachments.
- Impression material, mixing pad, spatula, modeling wax, aspirator tip/saliva ejector.

Laboratory stage
- Casting impressions.
- Making a cobalt chromium framework for the partial dentures.

Fourth visit (for chrome partials)

Note that this stage is not necessary for acrylic partial dentures.

- Trying the cobalt chromium framework and making minor adjustments, if necessary.
- Recording the shade of the teeth.
- Writing a detailed prescription (e.g. design of the denture, whether retainers are to be used, and shade) to accompany the impressions and occlusal record to be sent to the laboratory.

❶ The impression must be disinfected before sending to the laboratory.

Instruments and materials required
- Mirror, straight probe, tweezers.
- Shade guide, pliers, handpieces, a selection burs.
- Aspirator tip/saliva ejector.

Laboratory stage
- Adding teeth to the cobalt chromium framework.

Fifth visit
- Trying the partial dentures—checking the fit, retention, support, and appearance and making adjustments, if necessary.
- Writing a detailed prescription to accompany the trial dentures being sent to the laboratory.

❶ The impression must be disinfected before sending to the laboratory.

Instruments and materials required
- Mirror, straight probe, tweezers.
- Modelling wax, Willis bite gauge or a pair of dividers, wax knife, LeCron carver, heat source, shade guide.
- Aspirator tip/saliva ejector, articulating paper, and Miller forceps.

Laboratory stage
- Processing the dentures.

Sixth visit
- Fitting the dentures and checking.
- Instructing the patient on aftercare before discharging them.

Instruments and materials required
- Mirror, straight probe, tweezers.
- Handpieces and a selection of burs.
- Pressure indicator paste.
- Aspirator tip/saliva ejector, articulating paper, and Miller forceps.

Immediate dentures

Dentures are usually made after extraction wounds have healed and alveolar bone resorption has stabilized following extractions. However, if the patient has teeth to be extracted and there is a need to maintain appearance and function, an immediate denture will be the option.

Procedure

The procedures are the same as for normal dentures, except it is not possible to try them because the teeth will be still present. The denture is taken to the final stage before the extractions are performed and the denture fitted. The patient should be recalled soon afterwards for checking the extraction wound and the fit of the denture.

Instruments and materials required

- The nurse must prepare both prosthetic and surgical equipment ready for use when immediate dentures are to be fitted (see 📖 Full dentures, p.286 and 📖 Surgical extractions, p.300)
- Materials as for conventional dentures.

Aftercare for dentures

It is important to look after any new dentures. There are some easy instructions to follow:

- Dentures should be cleaned twice per day, and if necessary after eating.
- Dentures should be cleaned over a bowl of water or over a folded towel, in case they are dropped and damaged.
- A small to medium brush should be used to ensure that all areas can be cleaned.
- If solutions or fizzy denture cleaners are used, the manufacturer's instructions should be followed closely.
- Dentures should be taken out overnight and left in water. Bleaching products should not be used as they can damage the dentures.
- If the dentures are sore, then an appointment should be made with the surgery. The dentures should be worn prior to the appointment so that the painful areas are apparent.
- Care should be taken when eating hard foods such as apples. Some hard foodstuffs such as carrots and apples should be chopped before eating.

Implants

Dental implantology covers the replacement of a tooth or teeth with a permanent fixed prosthesis within either the mandible or the maxilla. Unlike a bridge, which relies on the teeth that remain, an implant is surgically placed into the bone. It could be said that this replaces the root(s) of a tooth that has been lost.

Using implants

Implants can be used to replace 1 missing tooth or, indeed, a full mandible or maxilla, but a thorough history and detailed examination should be carried out before any implant treatment is offered. Although tooth loss is not uncommon, it is important to establish how the tooth was lost because this could have contraindications on how the space is managed, and to check on bone density to make sure that the candidate is suitable.

Reasons for tooth loss

The main reasons for tooth loss include the following:
• Dental caries.
• Periodontal disease.
• Failure of endodontic treatment.
• Hypodontia—congenitally missing teeth.
• Trauma.

Each case presents the clinician with a different problem in relation to the choice and success of the implant, hence the need for a detailed history and examination.

Procedure

Although there are a wide range of implants available, they all rely on the process of osseo-integration, which can be described as the joining of the implant surface and the surrounding bone.

Following a full assessment an appointment will be made for the surgery.

Where the implant is to be placed, a small incision will be made in the gingiva. An area of bone will be removed, forming a small hole roughly the size of the implant. The implant is placed into the prepared area. Depending on the surrounding bone, a bone graft may be required.

The gingiva is then sutured back into place.

The type of implant system used will determine the requirements for future appointments; once healing has taken place, subsequent restorative procedures can begin.

Implant treatment is complex and requires time and experience to complete. Implant manufacturers sometimes run courses for the dental team, which can be of benefit to the dental nurse.

Root-canal treatment or therapy (RCT)

Endodontology covers the form, function, and health of the dental pulp and periradicular tissues. It encompasses many procedures, one of which is RCT.

Rationale

The dental pulp can be damaged by caries, trauma, periodontal disease, and operative dental procedures, which can lead to pulp death and bacterial infection. It is now known that the infecting bacteria remain within the pulp, producing toxins that leach out of the apical foramina and cause a periapical infection. When the pulp space is cleaned of all infecting material and sealed, so that bacteria cannot re-enter, the periapical lesion heals. Although a tooth is non-vital following RCT, it can function properly in the mouth because its periodontal attachment is healthy.

Aims of RCT

- To clean the pulp space of infected materials.
- To seal the pulp space to prevent re-infection from periapical or coronal directions.
- To maintain tooth function.

The stages of procedure

First visit

- Diagnosis and treatment planning.
- Administer local analgesia and isolate with a rubber dam.
- Gain access to the pulp space or root-canal system by drilling through the crown of the tooth.
- Remove pulpal debris.
- Disinfect root-canal system by irrigation.
- Clean and shape the root canal.
- Establish the correct length of the root—the working length by radiography and electronic methods.
- Inter-appointment medication.

Equipment and materials needed (first visit)

- Mirror and probe.
- Tweezers.
- Excavators.
- Handpieces and burs.
- Broaches (for removing vital tissue from the pulp and root-canal space).
- Files (for shaping root canals—hand-held or engine-driven).
- Spiral fillers (for placing dressings or medicaments within root canals).
- Spreaders and pluggers (used during filling or obturation of root canals).
- Syringes and needles (for irrigating root canals).
- Gates–Glidden burs (for enlarging root-canal openings or orifices).
- Safe-ended burs (for accessing pulp chamber safely).

- Electric pulp testers (for testing the vitality of a tooth).
- Electronic apex locators (for estimating the working length of root canals).
- Measuring blocks (for setting rubber rings or stoppers at correct points on the file).
- Irrigants (for cleaning and disinfecting root canals, such as sodium hypochloride [bleach]).
- Paper points.
- Medicaments (for dressing root canals between appointments, such as non-setting calcium hydroxide [Hypocal® and Reogan®]).
- Temporary restorative material.

Second visit
- Local analgesia and rubber dam.
- Remove temporary filling.
- Access pulp chamber and root canals.
- Irrigation and drying.
- Cone fit radiograph with gutta-percha in root canal.
- Obturation.
- Restoration of the tooth.

Equipment and materials needed (second visit)
- Mirror and probe.
- Tweezers.
- Excavators.
- Handpieces and burs.
- Irrigants.
- Syringes and needles.
- Measuring blocks.
- Paper points.
- Gutta-percha (GP) points.
- GP pluggers and spreaders.
- Sealer.
- Systems for obturating root canals, such as System B and Obtura.
- Permanent or temporary restorative material.

Colour coding of instruments

The size (diameter) and shape of the various instruments used inside root canals are important considerations.

Size

To facilitate accurate use, the handle carries the size imprinted at the top (e.g. 13, 20, and 23). In addition, a system of colour coding, related to tip diameters, is used.

It is the dental nurse's duty to hand over the instrument of correct size to the dentist during RCT. This system of colour coding is shown in Table 13.2.

Table 13.2 Colour coding of instruments

Colour	Tip diameter (mm)	Size
White	0.15	15
Yellow	0.20	20
Red	0.25	25
Blue	0.30	30
Green	0.35	35
Black	0.40	40

Shape

Because root canals become narrower from the crown (end) to the root (apex), the instruments used inside the root canals must have a similar shape. This change in diameter of an instrument is termed 'taper'. However, files made of nickel titanium (NiTi) have a different taper.

Because the tapers of NiTI files are greater than those of conventional files, these are called greater-taper (GT) files. A common shorthand is 'NiTi GT files'.

Methods of shaping root canals

There are several methods or protocols for shaping root canals, the most logical of which is the 'crown-down technique'. In this method, shaping the root canal begins by enlarging the coronal end first. Files with a larger diameter are used initially. In fact, Gates–Glidden burs might be used to enlarge the root-canal opening or orifice. As files are advanced into the root canal, smaller files are used.

▶ It is important for the nurse to know the method used so that the files can be handed down in the correct order. Colour coding the file handles makes it easier and safer for both the dentist and the nurse to select the correct-sized file.

Current safe practice is to use files only once and discard.

Irrigation of root canals

The purpose of irrigation is to clean and disinfect root canals while shaping them. The most effective irrigant is sodium hypochlorite (bleach). This is a very caustic material and only a 5% solution is used.

▶ Because of the harmful nature of sodium hypochlorite, every precaution must be taken to prevent spilling the liquid onto the patient's soft tissues and clothing, in addition to injection into periapical tissues. Most RCTs are carried out under rubber-dam isolation. Even with this precaution, copious aspiration must be used to take away safely the excess liquid during irrigation. The nurse must get the correct strength of solution, correct syringe and needle, aspirate efficiently, and be watchful during the whole procedure.

Estimation of the working length of root canals

The working length is the distance from a reference point on the crown (e.g. the incisal edge or tip of a cusp) to a point within the root canal at which the root filling ends. This end point in a mature tooth is an anatomical feature called the 'apical constriction' at which the root canal suddenly narrows. Beyond the apical constriction is periapical tissue.

The tried and tested method of establishing the correct working length of root canals is radiography. In this method, a rubber ring (stopper) is placed on the file and the file inserted into the root canal so that its tip is at the approximate position of the apical constriction and the rubber ring is aligned with the reference point selected (e.g. incisal edge). Then a radiograph is taken, processed, and viewed to confirm that the file is correctly placed, enabling the working length to be calculated.

> It is the nurse's duty to ensure that the rubber ring (stopper) is correctly placed at the set distance from the tip of the file (by use of a suitable measuring block), the file has not moved during radiography, and the x-ray film processor is working properly.

In the modern dental practice, electronic apex locators are used during initial placement of the file tip at the apical constriction. These are complicated electronic devices that indicate the position of the file tip in a user-friendly fashion.

> The nurse must ensure that the electronic apex locator is working properly, for example by checking that the battery is not low or dead.

Obturation of root canals

After cleaning and shaping root canals, elimination of any signs and symptoms of pulpal and periapical disease such as pain, swelling, discharging sinus, the root canals are obturated. The conventional method is to use GP cones with a sealer to obturate the root canals. Because the ready-to-use GP cones do not match the size and shape of individual root canals, several cones must be used, according to a set protocol. The largest and best-fitting GP cone that is used first is called the 'master GP cone' and subsequent cones placed alongside it in the root canal by use of a spreader are called 'accessory GP cones'.

If the whole procedure is carried out without warming the GP cones, the method is called 'cold lateral condensation'. If the GP cones are warmed (by a variety of ways using special equipment), the method is called 'warm condensation'.

There are a variety of methods and equipment available, such as Thermafil®, System B®, Obtura®, and Ultrafil®.

Recently, synthetic obturation materials have been introduced in place of GP (e.g. Real Seal® and Epiphany®).

> The nurse must ensure that the correct equipment and materials to be used are ready to hand, according to the protocol.

Shaping root canals with engine-driven or rotary instruments

The conventional method of shaping root canals has been superseded by the use of engine-driven instruments. However, this method is not new because rotary methods have been use before. What is new is the use of NiTi GT files. These files are very flexible and can be used in extremely curved canals. There is also the advantage of needing fewer file sizes. However, this type of file can cut dentine rapidly, leading to perforations and also fracture.

There are several brands, each with a unique protocol (e.g. Protaper® and System B®).

The nurse must ensure that they are familiar with the equipment and protocol used.

Surgical endodontics

Conventional RCT is non-surgical. However, in certain situations, surgery is used as an adjunct to eliminating periapical infection and sealing the root canals. In multi-rooted teeth it is possible that 1 root might not be easily treated by conventional methods, in which case the offending root can be resected, leaving the rest of the tooth in function.

The following are surgical endodontic procedures (see Chapter 14 for more details):
- Apicetomy.
- Incision and drainage of periapical abscesses.
- Furcation repair.
- Periapical curettage.
- Retrograde root filling.
- Root amputation.
- Root hemisection.

Concluding remarks

RCT used to be a time-consuming and tedious procedure. With the introduction of new equipment, materials, and techniques, it is no longer so. However, the goals of RCT remain the same: that is, to treat the diseases of the pulp and periapical tissues so that the offending tooth can remain in function. One has to be meticulous in carrying out the procedures to achieve a successful outcome.

Oral surgery

Extraction of erupted teeth

The removal of teeth is most commonly carried out under local anaesthesia. It can also be carried out under general anaesthesia, or a combination of sedation and local anaesthesia.

Stages during the procedure

- Ensure patient has followed all pre-operative instructions.
- Administer local aesthetic to the patient.
- The tooth socket is dilated using an elevator (extraction of erupted teeth can sometimes be carried out using just forceps especially if the tooth is mobile).
- The tooth is grasped around the crown using forceps and movement is applied to break the periodontal attachment.
- The tooth is removed from the socket.
- A gauze pack is placed over the socket and pressure is applied to help stop the bleeding.
- Postoperative advice is given to the patient.
- Gauze pack is removed and socket is checked to confirm bleeding has stopped.
- Patient is checked to ensure they are fit to leave.

Role of the dental nurse

- Collect the patient notes and identify the planned procedure.
- Prepare the clinical environment.
- Prepare the relevant instruments, materials, and equipment needed for the procedure, including PPE for the dental team and patient.
- Select and prepare the local anaesthetic and pass it to the dentist.
- Aspirate and retract the soft tissues to maintain a clear field of vision while the tooth is being removed.
- Pass the gauze pack to the dentist.
- Provide the patient with postoperative instructions.
- Provide the patient with some spare gauze packs to take home in case of bleeding.

Instruments and materials

- Mirror, straight probe, tweezers
- Aspirator tip
- Local anaesthetic cartridge, syringe, and needle
- Selection of elevators
- Extraction forceps
- Gauze packs
- Postoperative instruction sheet

Postoperative instructions

Following the procedure the dental nurse should give the patient the following postoperative instructions both verbally and in writing:
- Avoid rinsing today, because this will cause bleeding.
- Maintain a soft diet today — e.g. banana, egg, juice, pasta, and rice.

- Avoid very hot fluids.
- Warn the patient that they will experience numbness for a few hours, until the anaesthetic wears off.
- Rinse the wound with warm salt water four times a day for one week, starting tomorrow.
- Avoid alcohol and smoking for 48h to aid healing.
- Avoid strenuous exercise today.
- In the event of bleeding, bite firmly on the socket with a clean gauze pack for at least 30 mins.
- Provide a number to call if the patient has concerns or cannot control bleeding.

Removal of roots

Sometimes just the root of a tooth may be left behind in the jaw following the fracture or the loss of the crown (due to extensive caries or fracture) or fracture during extraction. If the root is easily accessible a procedure similar to that of the extraction of an erupted tooth can be used. The remaining tooth structures can be loosened using elevators, and then root forceps (which are narrower than standard forceps) can be used to remove the root.

Surgical extractions

Surgical extractions involve raising of a flap of gingiva with or without the removal of alveolar bone to gain access to the tooth or root. Conditions such as impacted lower 3rd molar teeth may require surgical extraction (this procedure may also require the impacted molars to be sectioned, to allow for their removal).

Surgical extractions can often be carried out under local anaesthetic, but will take longer to perform than a standard extraction.

Other reasons for surgical extraction include:
• Retained root following previous attempts at a tooth extraction.
• Partially erupted tooth.
• Retained deciduous tooth.
• Associated pathology (e.g. cysts).
• In order to perform orthodontic treatment, or to facilitate a prosthesis.

Stages during the procedure
• Ensure patient has followed all pre-operative instructions.
• Administer local aesthetic to the patient.
• A scalpel may be used to raise a gingiva flap to expose the tooth or overlying bone.
• Any overlying bone can be removed using a straight surgical handpiece and surgical bur.
• If tooth sectioning is required this can be done using a straight surgical handpiece and surgical bur (cool flow of saline required during use to prevent the build-up of heat from friction of the bur).
• The tooth or root is removed using a combination of elevators and forceps.
• The flap of gingiva is then placed back over the area and sutured back into position.
• A gauze pack is placed over the area and pressure is applied to help stop the bleeding.
• Postoperative advice is given to the patient.
• Gauze pack is removed and socket is checked to confirm bleeding has stopped.
• Patient is checked to ensure they are fit to leave.
• A further appointment is made for a review suture removal (unless dissolvable sutures have been used).

Role of the dental nurse
• Collect the patient notes and identify the planned procedure.
• Prepare the clinical environment.
• Prepare the relevant instruments, materials, and equipment needed for the procedure, including PPE for the dental team and patient.
• Select and prepare the local anaesthetic and pass it to the dentist.
• Aspirate and retract the soft tissues to maintain a clear field of vision while the tooth is being removed.
• Assist with the placement of sutures (aspirate, retract and cut sutures).
• Pass the gauze pack to the dentist.

- Provide the patient with postoperative instructions.
- Provide the patient with some spare gauze packs to take home in case of bleeding.
- Make a further appointment for the patient to return for the removal of sutures (unless dissolvable sutures have been used) and review.

Instruments and materials

- Mirror, straight probe, tweezers
- Local anaesthetic cartridge, syringe, and needle
- Surgical aspirator tip
- Sterile water for irrigation
- Periosteal elevator
- Cheek retractor
- Selection of elevators
- Extraction forceps
- Scalpel handle and blade
- Straight surgical handpiece and bur
- Suture needle and silk
- Needle holders and suture scissors
- Gauze packs
- Postoperative instruction sheet

Postoperative instructions

Following the procedure the dental nurse should give the patient the following postoperative instructions both verbally and in writing:
- Avoid rinsing today, because this will cause bleeding.
- Maintain a soft diet today — e.g. banana, egg, juice, pasta, and rice.
- Avoid very hot fluids.
- Warn the patient that they will experience numbness for a few hours until the anaesthetic wears off.
- Rinse the wound with warm salt water four times a day for one week, starting tomorrow.
- Avoid alcohol and smoking for 48h to aid healing.
- Avoid strenuous exercise today.
- In the event of bleeding, bite firmly on the socket with a clean gauze pack for at least 30mins.
- Advice on suture removal or dissolvable sutures.
- Advice on suitable medication in the event of pain/swelling.
- Provide a number to call if the patient has concerns or cannot control bleeding.

Other surgical procedures

Biopsies

A biopsy is a sample of tissue which is taken from a patient for histo-pathological examination. They are carried out to investigate and diagnose lesions, cysts or tumours that are found in the oral cavity.

Biopsies may be **incisional** (removal of part of the lesion) or **excisional** (removal of whole lesions) depending on the nature of the lesion, cyst, or tumour being investigated.

Operculectomy

During the eruption of a third molar tooth there is a flap of overlying gingiva (operculum) which normally degenerates until the whole occlusal surface has erupted. However, during eruption the operculum can remain on the occlusal surface and is bitten down on by the opposing tooth. This can cause swelling and inflammation which causes discomfort for the patient, and as the symptoms get worse, the patient may find it more difficult to clean the area.

Hot saline mouth washes, thorough cleaning, and antibiotics can be used to treat the area, however surgical intervention can be used to eliminate the problem. The flap can be removed under local anaesthetic, using a scalpel blade to cut away the flap. The remaining edges can then be cauterised to prevent bleeding.

Alveolectomy

The extraction of multiple teeth at the same time can leave the socket edges sitting proud of the alveolar bone. If a removable prosthesis is to be constructed for the patient, these bone edges can present a problem as the prosthesis will sit on top of them - this can be very uncomfortable. At the time of the extraction an **alveolectomy** can therefore be performed to remove the socket edges. Removal can be done using bone rongeurs (also known as bone 'nibblers') or a surgical handpiece and bur, to trim the socket edges.

Complications following surgical procedures

It is possible (no matter how much care is taken to ensure the appropriate preventative measures are taken) for complications to occur both during and after an extraction.

Haemorrhage (bleeding)

Primary and reactionary haemorrhage

During every extraction haemorrhage is a natural occurrence. This type of haemorrhage is called **primary haemorrhage** and normally stops within a few minutes following an extraction.

Haemostasis (arrest of bleeding) is achieved by placing a pressure pad (pressure applied to a sterile gauze placed over the area) for a few minutes.

Sometimes, although haemostasis was achieved following the extraction, bleeding can resume a few hours afterwards. This type of bleeding is called **reactionary haemorrhage**. It is usually caused by loss or disturbance of the blood clot (most often as a result of the patient not following the correct postoperative instructions). Haemostasis can be achieved by reapplication of a pressure pad, or by suturing together the edges of the socket.

A haemostatic drug (one which stops bleeding) such as adrenaline (epinephrine) can be used in conjunction with a pressure pad to help promote haemostasis. The drug can be applied to part of the pressure pad, or alternatively an absorbable pack can be placed into the socket and a pressure pad placed over the top.

Where reactionary haemorrhage has occurred, reinforcement of the postoperative instructions is advised.

Secondary haemorrhage

Secondary haemorrhage is seen much less commonly in the dental practice. It normally occurs 3-5 days after the procedure and can be caused by the formed blood clot not organizing properly due to disorders in patients such as haemophiliacs.

In general and major surgery secondary haemorrhage can occur 7–10 days after the operation, and is commonly due to infection.

Tooth fracture

Teeth that have been heavily restored, are grossly carious, or that have been root treated are more likely to fracture during extraction. There are no real preventative measures that can be taken, but the dental team can prepare by ensuring that the patient is pre-warned about the possibility of the fracture, and by making preparations to undertake a surgical procedure to remove the remaining section of the tooth.

Loss of a tooth

During an extraction a tooth may slip out of the grip of the forceps and become 'lost'. It could be that the tooth is dropped in the mouth and either aspirated by the quick-thinking dental nurse, swallowed, or inhaled by the patient. When a tooth disappears it must be looked for inside and outside the patient's mouth to establish where it is. It may be found on the patient or on the floor of the surgery, in which case the tooth can be dealt with as normal. Sometimes the patient is aware that they have swallowed something, and will be able to tell you. If the tooth has been swallowed, no further action is taken.

❶ If it is discovered that the tooth has been inhaled the patient must be referred to hospital, as an urgent operation will be required to remove it from the lung before it causes serious complications.

Perforation of the maxillary sinus

The roots of the upper teeth are very close to the floor of the maxillary sinus. During the extraction of an upper tooth the floor of the sinus may become perforated. In most cases the perforation will be small and no further action is required, because the perforation will be protected by a blood clot. However, if the perforation is larger it must be closed.

A perforation of this kind is called an **oral antral fistula** which means an unnatural communication between the oral cavity and the maxillary sinus.

An oral antral fistula can be detected by the appearance of bubbles in the socket when the patient blows their nose. Closure of these perforations is required to prevent infection in the sinus.

Small perforations can be closed by suturing the sides of the socket; but larger ones require coverage by a flap of mucosa, which is stretched and sutured over the perforation.

Infection

Loss of a blood clot from a socket can leave the walls of the socket bare, and as a result the socket can become inflamed an infected. This normally occurs 2-3 days following an extraction, and is called **localized osteitis (dry socket)**. This is a condition which is more commonly seen in patients who smoke or those with poor oral hygiene but can be seen in cases where the blood clot has been disturbed or lost; or where there is infection of the blood clot. The patient will return to the surgery complaining of acute throbbing pain in the quadrant where the tooth was extracted.

This is a condition which can be very painful, and patients may be quite distressed. Treatment of the infection and pain is given by syringing the socket to remove any debris and inserting a sedative dressing.

An analgesic drug is usually recommended to the patient, and reinforcement of the postoperative instructions is also advised.

Paediatric dentistry

The child as a patient

As a patient, the young child differs in several respects to older children and adults. The most important difference is that they will not have the understanding to cooperate with treatment or be logical about the need for a local anaesthetic (LA) or brushing their teeth. The parent or carer forms part of the 'paediatric triangle' with the clinician and child patient. The dental nurse has an important role in explaining and encouraging both child and parent to and from the dental chair and waiting room. During a dental examination or treatment, a child might also become distracted by instructions or conversations from more than one person and has a short attention span. This means that the dental nurse must be ready and willing to be flexible about dental procedures. For instance, if a child becomes uncooperative during restorative treatment, a temporary restoration might be needed.

Role of the dental nurse
- Meet and greet the child and parent/carer.
- Encourage the child to sit in the dental chair.
- Reassure the parent.
- Show the child the dental mirror, air, and suction.
- Use child-friendly language.
- Chart teeth present and carious teeth.
- Praise the child after treatment and give them a sticker.

Preventive dentistry for children

The main preventative approach for children is the use of fluoride tooth-paste. A pea-sized amount is appropriate and supervised brushing is recommended for young children. Parents can start brushing their children's teeth once deciduous teeth are present, by sitting the child on their lap both facing forwards and brushing with a small toothbrush and a pea-sized amount of children's (low-fluoride) toothpaste. For children <6 years of age, children's toothpaste with lower fluoride levels is recommended, unless the child has many carious teeth. After this age, children can use adult (high-fluoride) toothpaste and might no longer need to be supervised. After brushing, children should spit out and not rinse their mouths. Adolescents who have fixed orthodontic bands or removable appliances might also need a daily fluoride rinse as an extra preventative measure. Occasionally, topical fluoride can be applied to carious lesions in very young children if treatment is not possible.

Other preventative measures are diet modification, plaque removal, and fissure sealants. Children with a high risk of caries should be encouraged to ↓ the frequency of sugar snacks or drinks. If the infant goes to sleep with a bottle, this should be discouraged because the flow of saliva is ↓ and cannot protect the teeth.

Fissure sealants

Fissure sealants protect the deep pits and fissures of permanent teeth when a child is at risk of developing caries. This is usually the occlusal surface of the 1st permanent molar but can also include the buccal fissure of mandibular molars, the palatal fissure of maxillary molars, or palatal pits of maxillary incisors.

Stages during fissure sealant
- Isolate the tooth using a rubber dam or cotton-wool rolls.
- Remove the plaque from the tooth.
- Rinse the tooth.
- Etch, rinse, and dry the enamel.
- Place the fissure sealant onto the fissure(s) and light cure.
- Check the occlusion.

Box 15.1 Instruments and materials (fissure sealants)

- Rubber dam or cotton-wool rolls.
- Slow hand piece with prophy paste.
- Pumice and water in a dappen pot.
- Etch and applicator.
- Fissure sealant—this will start curing in natural light.
- Light cure unit and shield.

Fluoride varnish

Stages during application of fluoride varnish
- Apply a small amount of fluoride varnish to lesions.
- Instruct the child/parent not to brush the area until the next day.

Box 15.2 Instruments and materials (fluoride varnish)

- Fluoride varnish.
- Applicator brush.

Role of the dental nurse

- Prepare instruments and materials (Boxes 15.1 and 15.2).
- Assist the clinician during the procedure.
- Maintain a dry field.
- Assist the patient after the procedure.

Advice on oral hygiene for children, parents, and guardians

Regular brushing of teeth with fluoride toothpaste can prevent caries. Brushing should start when teeth first erupt into the mouth. Children should be encouraged to brush twice daily with a pea-sized amount of children's or adult toothpaste. Plaque-disclosing will help children and parents to brush effectively. Parents should supervise children until the child has the manual dexterity and understanding to brush each surface of each tooth themselves. Older children have sufficient manual dexterity to floss.

Stages during procedure
- Disclose the plaque with a disclosing tablet or solution.
- Show the child and parent areas of plaque.
- Show the child and parent the brushing technique.
- The child or parent should be able to demonstrate the brushing technique correctly when asked.
- Remove the plaque with a rubber cup/brush and slow hand piece.

Role of the dental nurse
- Prepare instruments and materials (see Box 15.3).
- Assist the clinician during the procedure.
- Assist the patient after the procedure.

Box 15.3 Instruments and materials (oral hygiene advice)

- Disclosing tablet or fluid.
- Petroleum jelly to protect lips.
- Hand-held face mirror for the child.
- Slow hand piece with a rubber cup or prophy brush.
- Prophylaxis paste in a dappen pot.

Restorative procedures for children

Restorative materials include composite, compomer, glass ionomer (cement), amalgam, and preformed metal crowns. The choice of material will be dictated by the extent of the carious lesion, the length of time before the tooth exfoliates, and the cooperation of the child. If caries is suspected or a small carious lesion is cleaned out, this can be filled with composite or glass ionomer and then fissure sealed. This is known as a 'preventive resin restoration'.

Stages during restoration

- Administer LA.
- Isolate the tooth using a rubber dam or cotton-wool rolls.
- Remove caries enamel and dentine.
- Matrix band, if the approximal surface is involved.
- Mix, place, cure, and carve the material of choice.
- Check the occlusion.
- Postoperative instructions for anaesthetic and restoration.

Stages during preventive resin restoration

- Directly investigate the fissure using a high-speed hand piece.
- Remove caries.
- Place the glass ionomer/composite lining, if necessary.
- Etch the enamel, rinse, and dry.
- Place the fissure sealant and use the light cure.
- Check the occlusion.

Role of the dental nurse

- Prepare instruments and materials (see Box 15.4).
- Operate suction.
- Mix the lining or restorative material, as required.
- Prepare the matrix band, if required.
- Assist the patient after the procedure.

Box 15.4 Instruments and materials (restorative procedures)

- Topical and LA agents.
- Rubber dam/cotton-wool rolls.
- Hand pieces and burs.
- Mixing pad and spatula.
- Calcium hydroxide lining, if required.
- Composite, glass ionomer, compomer, and amalgam.
- Matrix band and wedge.
- Occlusal paper to check the occlusion postoperatively.

Dental trauma in the child

Dental trauma in the child is a very distressing experience for both child and parent. Some kind of dental trauma is experienced by ~30% of children. These injuries include:

- Avulsed teeth—teeth that are knocked completely out.
- Fractured teeth.
- Teeth moved out of position—forced upwards, outwards, inwards, or backwards.
- Fractures of the root.
- Fractures of the supporting bone.

During a person's lifetime, they will have 2 sets of teeth. Up to 6 years of age there will be the deciduous dentition. After 6 years of age the dentition is mixed, with both deciduous and permanent teeth present. At approximately 15–16 years of age all deciduous teeth will have been lost, leaving the permanent teeth.

Trauma to the dentition can occur during all these stages.

Trauma to the deciduous dentition commonly occurs at 18–40 months of age. This is when the toddler is exploring their world and there will be numerous falls and collisions, which can result in trauma to the dentition.

Teenage boys are twice as likely to suffer trauma to the permanent teeth as teenage girls. The teeth most commonly affected are the upper incisors owing to sports accidents and fights.

Clinical evaluation for all trauma situations

Medical history

A medical history is taken is to rule out any problems that might influence the treatment, such as heart or bleeding problems and loss of consciousness.

Dental history

How, when, and where the injury took place. 'When' is important because the time of injury influences the prognosis. 'Where' is important in relation to tetanus prophylaxis.

Extraoral examination

To see whether there are any facial lacerations or bruising and ensure no mandibular or zygomatic fractures. Limited opening, anterior open bite, and malocclusion indicate a fractured condyle.

Intraoral examination

The alveolus is palpated to detect fracture. Soft-tissue lacerations are cleaned and explored for foreign bodies. Most intraoral lacerations will heal by themselves, although some must be sutured.

Radiographic examination

Determines the extent and type of damage. This is particularly helpful for root fractures, which cannot be detected by visual examination of the mouth.

Avulsion

Dental avulsion is defined as the complete displacement of a tooth out of its socket.

Hopefully, the tooth will have been stored in an acceptable medium to prevent dehydration, as follows:
- Milk.
- Saline.
- Contact lens solution.
- Water—as a last resort.

Deciduous tooth

An avulsed deciduous tooth is not usually re-implanted because of possible damage to the developing permanent tooth.

Permanent tooth

Children with an avulsed tooth will usually attend as an emergency, with a parent, very soon after the incident. The treatment for an avulsed permanent tooth is to re-implant it in its socket.

Stages during procedure

- Assess the tooth to determine whether it is suitable for re-implanting.
- Administer a LA.
- Clean the socket of blood clots with saline.
- The tooth is picked up by the crown and gently inserted into the socket.
- The labial and palatal/lingual bony plates are gently compressed.
- A flexible, functional splint is placed for 7–10 days.* This is usually thin orthodontic wire bent into the shape of the arch and attached to the teeth by composite material. If an alveolar fracture is present, a rigid splint is placed for 4–6 weeks.

* High-tensile fishing wire can be used as an effective functional splint and is easier to apply than orthodontic wire.

Role of the dental nurse

- Be friendly, cheerful, and confident.
- Reassure and calm the patient.
- Calm and reassure the parent that their child is in good hands.
- Collect or make new notes for the patient.
- Prepare the clinical environment.
- Prepare the relevant instruments, materials, and equipment needed for the reimplantation (see Box 15.5).
- Retract the soft tissue and aspirate to maintain as dry a field as possible during reimplantation.
- Pass the splinting material to the dentist and universal orthodontic pliers, if wire is the splinting material of choice.
- Pass the acid etch material, bond, and composite to the dentist in sequence.
- Pass the curing light to the dentist.

Box 15.5 Instruments and materials (avulsion)

- Mirror, straight probe, tweezers, wire cutters, flat plastic, orthodontic universal pliers, composite kit, and curing light.
- LA cartridge, syringe, and a short needle.
- Dappen pots for acid etch and bond.

Aftercare instructions

After re-implantation the patient should be given a mouth rinse. The patient and parent are instructed to keep the mouth as clean as possible but avoid strenuous brushing of the teeth. Chlorhexidine mouthwash and, possibly, an antibiotic are prescribed. A review appointment is made in 1 week.

Tooth fracture: deciduous dentition

Crown fractures in the dentition account for ~33% of injuries to deciduous teeth and ~75% of injuries to the permanent teeth (Fig. 15.1).

Classifications of fractures are descriptive:
- Fracture of the enamel only.
- Fracture of the enamel and dentine.
- Fractures involving enamel, dentine, and pulp.

Treatment

Treatment of an enamel-only fracture
Smooth the fractured edges, leave, or restore with composite.

Treatment of a fracture of the enamel and dentine
Cover the dentine with a glass ionomer cement, review within a few weeks, and restore with composite.

Treatment of a more complex fracture involving the pulp
There are several options, as follows:
- Direct pulp capping—for small pulpal exposures.
- Pulpotomy—partial removal of the pulp.
- Extraction.

Pulpectomy
Pulpectomy (total removal of the pulp) can damage the permanent successor, especially in incisors. Pulpectomy is usually only carried out in the deciduous dentition on dead abscessed teeth or hyperaemic dying pulps.

Stages during pulpotomy procedure
- See Box 15.6 for appropriate instruments and materials.
- Administer a LA.
- Apply a rubber dam.
- Dry the field.
- Remove 1–2mm of pulp tissue.
- Apply ferric sulphate to the pulp.
- Seal the area with zinc oxide or glass ionomer cement.

Box 15.6 Instruments and materials (pulpotomy procedure)

- Mirror, straight probe, flat plastic, relevant hand pieces, and burs.
- LA cartridges and syringe.
- Rubber dam kit.
- Mixing pad.
- Glass ionomer and zinc oxide cement.
- Ferric sulphate.
- Setting and non-setting calcium hydroxide.
- Extraction forceps.

Aftercare instructions
Review after 1 week to see whether the patient is symptom-free.

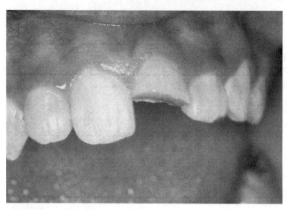

Fig. 15.1 Typical tooth fracture.

Tooth fracture: permanent dentition

Treatment

Treatment of an enamel-only fracture
The edges are smoothed and fracture restored with composite.

Treatment of a fracture of the enamel and dentine
The dentine is coated with a protective layer, such as glass ionomer cement, to form a temporary 'bandage'. A final composite restoration is placed some weeks later.

Treatment of a more complex fracture involving the pulp
The aim is to maintain a viable pulp so that root formation can be completed.

Treatment options are as follows:
- Direct capping of the pulp—used for a recent small pulp exposure and involves covering the exposure with a layer of setting calcium hydroxide before restoring with composite material.
- Cvek pulpotomy—minimal removal of pulp material that is performed on pulp exposures >2mm. A round bur is used to remove 1–2mm of pulpal tissue. The pulp is then covered with a layer of non-setting calcium hydroxide, which is sealed with glass ionomer cement.
- Deeper cervical pulpotomy—for an exposure >2 hours. The procedure is similar to that described for a Cvek pulpotomy, except that more pulpal tissue is removed.

The final restoration will be composite material of a suitable shade.

Stages during procedure

Pulp capping
- Administer a LA.
- Place a rubber dam.
- Dry the field.
- Smooth fracture edges.
- Place a layer of setting calcium hydroxide over the exposure.
- Restore with composite material.

Cvek pulpotomy
- Administer a LA.
- Place a rubber dam.
- Dry the field.
- Remove 1–2mm of pulp tissue.
- Place a layer of non-setting calcium hydroxide over the pulp.
- Seal the area with glass ionomer cement.

Deeper cervical pulpotomy
The stages are similar to those described for a Cvek pulpotomy, except that more pulpal tissue is removed.

Pulpectomy
- Administer a LA.
- Place a rubber dam.
- Dry the field.
- The pulp chamber is opened by use of a round bur.
- Pulp fragments are cleaned out using files and washed with saline.
- Dry.
- Insert non-setting calcium hydroxide—usually the preparation comes in a syringe. Alternatively, a mixture of iodoform paste and non-setting calcium hydroxide can be inserted.
- Ledermix paste can be used as an alternative to calcium hydroxide/iodoform paste.
- Seal the area with glass ionomer or zinc oxide cement.

Role of the dental nurse
- Collect or make new notes for the patient.
- Prepare the clinical environment.
- Prepare the relevant instruments, materials, and equipment needed for the treatment of tooth fractures (see Box 15.7).
- Aspirate to maintain as dry a field as possible.
- Pass the relevant materials and instruments to the dentist, as requested.

Box 15.7 Instruments and materials (tooth fractures)

- Mirror, straight probe, and flat plastic.
- LA cartridge and syringe.
- Rubber dam kit.
- Relevant hand pieces and burs.
- Root-canal files.
- Syringe of saline.
- Mixing pad.
- Spatula.
- Glass ionomer cement.
- Non-setting and setting calcium hydroxide or a mixture of iodoform paste and non-setting calcium hydroxide.

Aftercare instructions
The patient should take paracetamol in case of pain postoperatively. Review after 1 week to see whether the patient is symptom-free.

Other common dental traumas

Tooth displacement (luxation)
Luxation involves the displacement of a tooth labially, lingually, or laterally.

Deciduous dentition
Treatment of labial luxation of a deciduous tooth is extraction, to avoid damage to the permanent tooth. With other luxation injuries, it might be possible to splint the tooth back into position with resin-modified glass ionomer cement. The splint is removed after 10 days. If the tooth is extruded, it is extracted.

Permanent dentition
The tooth is usually repositioned, under a LA, and splinted for 2–3 weeks with a semi-rigid splint. A post-treatment radiograph should be taken to check positioning. For an extrusive luxation only, the tooth is repositioned and splinted with a semi-rigid splint for 7–14 days.

Tooth intrusion
The tooth is pushed up into the socket, crushing the periodontal ligament, rupturing blood vessels, fracturing the alveolar bone, and, possibly, damaging the developing permanent tooth if the injury is in the deciduous dentition.

Deciduous dentition
Usually the intruded tooth will spontaneously erupt over a 2–3 month period. If not, it should be extracted. Severely intruded teeth are extracted immediately.

Permanent dentition
Permanent incisors intruded <3mm usually reposition themselves over time.

Intrusions of 3–6mm might have to be orthodontically extruded.

For intrusions >6mm, the tooth should be surgically repositioned, a pulpectomy performed, and the root canal filled with calcium hydroxide.

Role of the dental nurse
• Collect or make new notes.
• Prepare the clinical environment.
• Prepare the relevant instruments, materials, and equipment for possible extraction of deciduous teeth.
• Prepare the relevant instruments for possible root-canal treatment.
• Pass the instruments to the dentist, as required.

Dental concussion
Quite often there can be injury to a tooth that results in no displacement or tooth mobility.

Deciduous dentition
Radiographs are taken to exclude root fracture. No other treatment is required. Parents must be cautioned that the colour of the tooth might darken because there is a possibility of damage to a blood vessel. If this occurs, the pulp of the tooth will have undergone necrosis (tissue death). The treatment is root-canal therapy, extraction, or regular monitoring until exfoliation.

A pink tooth indicates internal resorption.

Permanent dentition

Radiographs are taken to exclude root fracture. If mobile, the tooth is splinted for 7–10 days. There must be regular reviews for vitality testing.

Root fracture

Root fractures occur in 7% of dental injuries. Usually they involve the anterior teeth.

Root fractures are classified by position, as follows:
• Apical 1/3.
• Middle 1/3.
• Coronal 1/3.

Deciduous dentition

If the tooth is not excessively mobile or infected, the fractured root can be left for natural exfoliation. If the tooth is mobile, the coronal part can be extracted and the rest left to exfoliate.

Permanent dentition

Most root fractures are horizontal. The fracture has to be reduced and immobilized with a rigid splint for 8 weeks to facilitate healing of the dentine and cementum. Radiographs are taken at 6-month intervals to monitor healing.

Stages during procedure
• Administer a LA.
• Manual reduction of the root fracture.
• Immobilization by rigid splint to adjacent teeth.
• Splint removal after 8 weeks.
• Radiographic review every 6 months.

Aftercare instructions

A chlorhexidine mouthwash is given to the patient, with instructions to keep the mouth as clean as possible but avoiding strenuous brushing.

Instruments and materials

These are similar to those used for routine splinting (see Box 15.5).

Orthodontics

Introduction: orthodontics

Orthodontics is a specialist branch of dentistry concerned with the correction of abnormalities of tooth position, known as 'malocclusion'. Treatment commonly involves straightening crooked teeth, closing gaps, and correction of protruding teeth. Orthodontics is most frequently undertaken in adolescent children (12–16 years old) but can be performed in any age group.

Reasons for orthodontic treatment

- Improvement in appearance—orthodontics can be undertaken alone or in conjunction with other branches of dentistry to improve facial and dental appearance.
- Psychological benefits—patients presenting with abnormalities of tooth position (malocclusion) can be subjected to teasing and bullying and might have a decreased quality of life. Orthodontic treatment can improve their self-esteem and quality of life.
- Improvement in dental health—the presence of straight, well-aligned teeth helps ensure effective plaque control. However, ideal dental alignment neither causes nor prevents dental caries or periodontal disease. Nevertheless, orthodontic treatment in certain situations can prevent dental disease in conjunction with patients who practise good oral hygiene routines.
- Aiding other dental or minor oral surgical treatment—orthodontics can be undertaken to enable other dental treatment (e.g. replacement of absent teeth with dental implants) by movement of adjacent teeth, thus creating sufficient space. Unerupted teeth, such as maxillary canines or central incisors, might require minor oral surgery to uncover them before their alignment. The oral surgery procedure used is commonly referred to as an 'expose and bond' which uncovers the teeth/tooth before their alignment.
- Combined orthodontic–surgical approach—patients with severe jaw (skeletal) discrepancies require orthodontic treatment in combination with jaw (orthognathic) surgery. Such combined treatment ensures optimal improvement in both facial and dental appearance, in addition to ↑ stability of the final result.

Cause of malocclusion

There are many causes of malocclusion that a dental nurse may come across, especially in an orthodontic environment. Some of these are genetic in nature whilst others which are less common are acquired:
- Abnormal jaw size (genetic):
  - Maxilla too big or too small.
  - Mandible too big or too small.
  - Combination of both.
- Supernumerary teeth (genetic).
- Missing teeth known as hypodontia (genetic or acquired).
- Early tooth loss (acquired).
- Sucking habits (acquired).
- Crowding (genetic).

Orthodontic classifications

Orthodontic classifications are a way of describing the different aspects of a malocclusion. In general, classification is divided into skeletal ('jaw') and dental ('incisor and molar') relationships. The skeletal relationship is a very important factor in determining the dental relationship.

Skeletal relationship

This describes how the upper (maxilla) and lower (mandible) jaws relate to one another. There are 3 different types of skeletal relationship:

- Class I (normal)—the maxilla is just forward of the mandible, giving a well-balanced facial profile and a class I incisor and molar relationship.
- Class II—the maxilla is too far forward of the mandible, giving rise to a class II incisor and molar relationship.
- Class III—the maxilla is behind the mandible, giving rise to a class III incisor and molar relationship.

Dental relationship

Incisor classifications

- Class I—the upper incisors are just forward of the lower incisors. This results in a normal overjet (horizontal projection of the upper incisors over the lower incisors) and overbite (vertical overlap of the upper incisors over the lower incisors) of 2–4mm.
- Class II—there are 2 types of class II incisor relationship:
  - Class II division 1—the upper incisors protrude forward, resulting in an ↑ overjet.
  - Class II division 2—the upper central incisors lean backward and the overjet is usually ↓ with an ↑ overbite.
- Class III— a 'reverse overjet' where the lower incisor teeth protrude too far forward of the upper incisor teeth

Molar relationship

- Class I—the upper 1st molar occludes just forward of the lower 1st molar.
- Class II—the upper 1st molar occludes too far forward of the lower 1st molar.
- Class III—the upper 1st molar occludes behind the lower 1st molar.

Removable appliances

A removable orthodontic appliance is one that can be removed by the patient for cleaning and is not connected to the teeth in any way. For tooth movement to occur a force must act on a tooth for at least 6 hours; consequently, patients are usually advised to wear removable appliances on a full-time basis. Removable appliances 'tip' the teeth rather than a fixed appliance that creates full tooth movement therefore they use less force than fixed appliances.

General components

Removable appliances have 4 main parts; these components can be remembered by the acronym 'ARAB':
- **A**ctive components—the parts used to move teeth, through the application of a force, which can be produced by springs or screws, for example.
- **R**etentive components—the parts used to hold the appliance in the mouth. Stainless steel (Adam's) clasps are typically used.
- **A**nchorage—the resistance to unwanted tooth movement. The application of a force to produce tooth movement always results in an equal-and-opposite force being generated and, as such, it is important that this force is resisted. This is achieved by ensuring the acrylic contacts as many teeth as possible.
- **B**ase plate—acrylic that links all the components together; it covers the palate and is made from self-cure acrylic.

Reasons for a removable appliance

The removable appliance is no longer considered suitable for complete treatment in most cases because of the excellent control of tooth movement by fixed appliances. Nevertheless, removable appliances can be used with fixed appliances; e.g. to prevent the patient from biting off the brackets from their lower incisors, in the case of an ↑ overbite.

Limitations

- Only limited tooth movement is possible.
- Very dependent on patient cooperation because of their removable nature.
- Require manufacture in a laboratory.
- Interfere with both speech and chewing in the short term.

First visit

- Full orthodontic examination is carried out.
- X-rays will be taken to ensure that all teeth are present and will also ensure that any missing teeth or supernumerary teeth are identified prior to treatment starting.
- Alginate impressions will be taken prior to treatment starting for study models.
- Photographs will be taken for reference.

Role of the dental nurse

- Collect patient notes and identify the planned procedure.
- Prepare the clinical environment.
- Prepare the relevant instruments, materials and equipment needed for the procedure including PPE for the dental team and patient (Box 16.1).
- Assist with and record orthodontic charting as necessary.
- Select appropriate impression trays, apply tray adhesive, and attach handle.
- Mix required amount of alginate impression material, load into tray and pass to dentist.
- Monitor and reassure the patient while the impression material is in their mouth.
- Disinfect impressions and place into a plastic bag.
- Ensure lab card is completed and liaise with reception to arrange a further appointment for the patient.

Box 16.1 Instruments and materials (removable appliances, first visit)

- Mirror, straight probe, tweezers.
- Impression trays, tray handles, tray adhesive, alginate, room temperature water, mixing spatula, mixing bowl, water measuring cup, modelling wax, heat source.
- Laboratory bag and card.
- Photographic mirror.
- Photographic cheek retractors.

Second visit

This is normally a visit to discuss the treatment that will be carried out and therefore is not usually long in duration. At this appointment the orthodontist will discuss the planned treatment with the patient. Alginate impressions may also be taken at this visit for the removable appliance to be made; if this is the case the role of the dental nurse will include aspects of the first visit in relation to impression taking.

Role of the dental nurse

- Collect patient notes and study models and radiographs.
- Prepare the clinical environment.
- Prepare the relevant instruments, materials and equipment needed for the procedure including PPE for the dental team and patient (Box 16.2).
- Assist the dentist with the taking of photographs.
- Select appropriate impression trays, apply tray adhesive, and attach handle.
- Monitor and reassure the patient during the treatment.
- Disinfect impressions and place into a plastic bag.
- Ensure lab card is completed and liaise with reception to arrange a further appointment for the patient.

Third visit

During this visit, the appliance will be fitted. This will involve the orthodontist trying the appliance in the patient's mouth. When the orthodontist is happy the patient will be given a hand mirror and asked to take the appliance in and out. The dental nurse may also be asked to instruct the patient on how to care for the appliance in relation to cleaning and general looking after of the appliance (see 📖 Care of appliances, p.340).

Role of the dental nurse
- Collect patient notes and study models, radiographs, and orthodontic appliance.
- Prepare the clinical environment.
- Prepare the relevant instruments, materials, and equipment needed for the procedure (Box 16.3) including PPE for the dental team and patient.
- Monitor and reassure the patient during the treatment.

- Pass appropriate instruments during the procedure.

Subsequent appointments will be arranged for the appliance to be checked and, where necessary, adjusted.

Retainers

Following orthodontic treatment, a period of retention is necessary to prevent the teeth from moving back towards their original malocclusion ('relapse'). Retainers can either resemble the typical removable appliance or more commonly consist of a softer, clear plastic, known as an 'Essix retainer'.

Fixed appliances

A fixed orthodontic appliance or brace that is fixed to the teeth, sometimes referred to as 'train tracks'

Background

Fixed orthodontic appliances are nowadays used to perform the majority of orthodontic treatment because they give precise 3-dimensional tooth movement. Fixed appliances cause bodily movement of teeth as opposed to 'tipping' teeth in to position. Teeth are moved through the alveolar bone to the desired position by the forces exerted by the fixed appliance directly on the tooth. Treatment with fixed appliances takes about 18 months, depending on the severity of the malocclusion. Throughout treatment, patients are usually seen at intervals of 6 weeks, as they progress through stages of treatment. In some cases teeth may need to be extracted to create enough room for tooth movement to take place.

General components

Fixed appliances consist of several components which all work together

- Bands—orthodontic bands can be placed on molar teeth instead of brackets; e.g. if headgear is being used. They are cemented with either glass ionomer cement or composite resin.
- Brackets—bonded, with composite resin, to the labial/buccal surface of the incisors, canines, and premolars. They are usually made of stainless steel, although clear plastic alternatives are gaining in popularity with adults.
- Archwire—during the initial stages of treatment, flexible archwires that exert light forces on the teeth are used, e.g. nickel–titanium (NiTi). In the later stages of treatment, stiffer archwires that exert stronger forces on the teeth are used, e.g. stainless steel (S/S). Archwires are available in 2 different shapes:
  - Round—used during the initial stages of treatment to move the crowns of teeth.
  - Rectangular—used towards the end stages of treatment to move the crown and root.
- Ligatures—these are used to hold the archwire in the bracket and can be elastic or stainless steel. Elastic ligatures are available in a variety of colours and must be changed at each appointment. More recently, self-ligating brackets, which include built-in metal shutters, have been developed to avoid the need for elastic ligatures.

Stages of treatment

- Initial stage—straightening the teeth. NiTi archwires are used (initially round and then rectangular archwires, see Fig. 16.1) because of their flexible nature. This stage of treatment is usually completed within 4–6 months.
- Intermediate stage—could include the use of round S/S archwires, during which teeth might need to be moved along the archwire by use of either NiTi springs or elastic chain.
- Final stage—involves the use of rectangular S/S archwires to achieve the best position for the crowns and roots of the teeth and final occlusion. When both the patient and orthodontist are happy with the

result, the fixed appliance is '*debonded*', by removing the composite adhesive from the teeth. The patient then receives either a bonded retainer which is fixed to the teeth or a removable *retainer*, to ensure the teeth remain straight while the bone and gingiva firm to the new tooth positions. On occasion both fixed and removable retainers can be used when 1 arch has a bonded retainer and the other arch has a removable retainer.

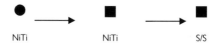

NiTi   NiTi   S/S

Fig. 16.1 Archwire progression, in terms of both shape and material, during treatment with a fixed appliance.

First visit
- Full orthodontic examination is carried out
- X-rays will be taken to ensure that all teeth are present and will also ensure that any missing teeth or supernumerary teeth are identified prior to treatment starting.
- Alginate impressions will be taken prior to treatment starting for study models.
- Photographs will be taken for reference.

Role of the dental nurse
- Collect patient notes and identify the planned procedure.
- Prepare the clinical environment.
- Prepare the relevant instruments, materials, and equipment needed for the procedure including PPE for the dental team and patient (Box 16.4).
- Assist with and record orthodontic charting as necessary.
- Assist the dentist with the taking of photographs.
- Select appropriate impression trays, apply tray adhesive, and attach handle.
- Mix required amount of alginate impression material, load into tray, and pass to dentist.
- Monitor and reassure the patient while the impression material is in their mouth.
- Disinfect impressions and place in to a plastic bag.
- Ensure lab card is completed and arrange a further appointment for the patient.

> **Box 16.4 Instruments and materials (fixed appliances, first visit)**
>
> - Mirror, straight probe, tweezers.
> - Impression trays, tray handles, tray adhesive, alginate, room temperature water, mixing spatula, mixing bowl, water measuring cup modelling wax, heat source.
> - Laboratory bag and card.
> - Photographic mirror.
> - Photographic cheek retractors.

Second visit: treatment planning visit

This is normally a visit to discuss the treatment that will be carried out and therefore is not usually long in duration. At this appointment the orthodontist will discuss the planned treatment with the patient. At this stage the orthodontist will decide if any extractions are necessary to make room for the movement of the teeth. If this is the case the orthodontist will refer the patient to their General Dental Practitioner for this to be carried out before orthodontic treatment is commenced.

Role of the dental nurse
- Collect patient notes, study models, and radiographs.
- Prepare the clinical environment.
- Prepare the relevant instruments, materials and equipment needed for the procedure including PPE for the dental team and patient (Box 16.5).

Box 16.5 Instruments and materials (fixed appliances, second visit)

- Mirror, straight probe, tweezers.
- Study models.
- Radiographs.

Third visit: placement of separators

During this visit and prior to the orthodontic bands being placed a small space needs to be created around the molar teeth. This will allow the bands to be placed.

Role of the dental nurse
- Collect patient notes, study models, and radiographs.
- Prepare the clinical environment.
- Prepare the relevant instruments, materials, and equipment needed for the procedure including PPE for the dental team and patient (Box 16.6).
- Assist the dentist.
- Monitor and reassure the patient during the treatment.

Box 16.6 Instruments and materials required (fixed appliances, third visit)

- Mirror, straight probe, tweezers.
- Separating pliers.
- Separators.

Aftercare
When the separators have been placed the patient may feel some discomfort whilst the space is created for the bands. Questions relating to the provision of pain relief should be referred to the orthodontist.

Fourth visit: placement of orthodontic bands and or brackets

- Orthodontic bands selected.
- Tried on the appropriate molar teeth and seated into position with a band seater.

- Once the dentist is happy with the fit the bands are removed with the band remover.
- Molar teeth cleaned and washed.
- Material mixed and loaded into the bands.
- Bands fitted in to position with band seater.
- Excess cement removed.

Role of the dental nurse

- Collect patient notes, study models, and radiographs.
- Prepare the clinical environment.
- Prepare the relevant instruments, materials and equipment needed for the procedure including PPE for the dental team and patient (Box 16.7).
- Aspirate when the teeth are being cleaned.
- Pass the appropriate instruments to the dentist.
- Mix the appropriate material when indicated by the dentist.
- Monitor and reassure the patient during the treatment.

Some orthodontists may also decide at this visit to cement the orthodontic brackets on to the teeth. Depending on the material selected will depend on the dental nurse's role.

Box 16.7 Instruments and materials (fixed appliances, fourth visit)

- Mirror, straight probe, tweezers.
- Band seater, band remover.
- Mixing spatula, wax pad, glass Ionomer powder, distilled water, measuring spoon flat plastic instrument.
- Orthodontic bands.

If cementing brackets the following will also be required:
- Light wire and/or Weingart's pliers.
- Ligature cutters.
- Distal-end cutters.
- Amalgam plugger or archwire tucker.
- Dental mirror.
- Mosquito forceps.

Aftercare

See 📖 Care of appliances, p.340.

Subsequent appointments

Patients visit the orthodontist every 4–6 weeks to have wires changed and various adjustments made to the appliance. This continues over a long period of time until the orthodontist is satisfied that the teeth are in the correct position. The patient will attend the surgery for a debond. During this procedure the fixed appliance is removed along with the bands from the teeth.

Any adhesive material is removed from the teeth by using a slow hand piece and *tungsten carbide bur*. An impression/s will be taken and a retainer made by the laboratory which will prevent the teeth from moving.

Functional appliances

Definition

An orthodontic appliance that is used to alter the growth of the jaws using the muscles of mastication and facial muscles. Functional appliances differ significantly from other removable appliances, which rely on forces produced by springs or screws to move teeth.

Background

- Functional appliances work best if treatment is timed to coincide with the pubertal growth spurt; this occurs at ~10–12 years in ♀ and ~11–14 years in ♂.
- Similar to removable appliances, functional appliances are made by use of study models, with alginate impressions and a special wax bite registration.
- Similar to removable appliances, to produce excellent results functional appliances must be worn on a full-time basis. Their removal for eating, contact sports, swimming, and cleaning of teeth and appliances is acceptable, however.

▶ Timing of treatment and patient motivation are ∴ very important factors in the success of treatment.

Indications

Functional appliances are very popular for correction of class II division 1 incisor relationships, in which the overjet is pronounced.

Types of functional appliance

Removable functional appliances

Most functional appliances are removable; the most popular of these in the UK is the twin-block appliance. The twin block consists of separate upper and lower appliances that are designed to come together in such a manner that they hold the mandible forward.

The advantage of this type of appliance is that it does not rely on patient compliance. However, associated problems include the risk of fracture of the appliance and ↑ plaque deposits on and around the teeth.

Mode of action

All functional appliances, whether fixed or removable, have a very similar mode of action; treatment changes are typically skeletal and dental in nature and might include the following:
- Temporary acceleration of mandibular growth.
- Temporary restraint of maxillary growth.
- Backward tipping ('retroclination') of upper incisors.
- Forward tipping ('proclination') of lower incisors.
- Control of molar eruption.
- Occlusal plane changes.

Functional appliance treatment usually takes 9–12 months. However, similar to all removable appliances, functional appliances cannot produce controlled movement of individual teeth; consequently, fixed appliances are often placed soon after treatment with functional appliances, to settle the buccal occlusion and detail the final result.

Limitations

Limitations of functional appliances are generally similar to those of removable appliances Alternatives to the use of functional appliances for class II correction includes the use of intermaxillary elastics and headgear; the success of these methods also depends on excellent patient motivation.

Extraoral traction 'headgear'

Definition

Headgear can be used to apply an extraoral force to either produce tooth movement ('extraoral traction') or prevent tooth movement ('extraoral anchorage'). Headgear can be fitted to either removable or fixed appliances.

Headgear components

Facebow

The facebow consists of an inner bow (which slots into a tube on either the fixed or the removable appliance) and outer bow (for attachment of a head cap or neckstrap).

Headcap or neckstrap

This component links the outer facebow to the head or neck and usually has an elastic component for delivering the force needed to either prevent or move the molar teeth.

Safety features

At least 2 safety features should be included in the headgear design, to limit the risk of injury. Recommended features include the following:
- Locking facebow—to prevent the facebow from becoming detached from the fixed or removable appliance.
- Additional cervical neckstrap
- Spring mechanisms—which release if excessive force is applied, preventing recoil or catapult of the facebow.

Fitting headgear

Headgear can be fitted to soldered tubes on removable appliances or, more usually, directly to bands on the upper 1st molars. Before discharging the patient, he/she must be able to fit and remove the headgear.

Indications

Typically, headgear is used in skeletal class II patterns associated with class II division 1 or 2 incisor relationships for 2 reasons, as follows:
- Extraoral anchorage—to prevent molar teeth from coming forwards after space is created by dental extraction of, e.g. the premolar teeth. Patients need only wear this type of headgear during bedtime hours (8–10 hours/day).
- Extraoral traction—to move the molar teeth backwards to create more space in the dental arch or relieve anterior dental crowding. Patients must wear the headgear for longer periods of time to achieve this backward movement of teeth (12–14 hours/day).

The decision as to whether anchorage or traction is needed depends on the degree of overjet and amount of crowding in the arch; a greater need for space might ensure extraoral traction is needed.

Limitations

- Poor cooperation—the major problem with headgear use, because most patients only achieve 50% of the expected wear. Cooperation might be improved by asking the patient to keep a chart of the number of hours they wear the headgear each day and encouragement at each recall visit.
- Injury—very rare as a result of wearing headgear, but usually from spontaneous detachment of the headgear at night or recoil of the headgear onto the face during attempted removal. For this reason, the inclusion of safety components is very important.

Instructions

Providing instructions before and after headgear insertion is important to improve patient cooperation and, more importantly, to ↓ the risk of head-gear-related injury. The following are important instructions to include:
- Wear the headgear for the recommended time.
- Keep a headgear calendar.
- Bring the headgear to each clinic visit.
- If the headgear falls out at night, return to the clinic as soon as convenient. Meanwhile, stop wearing the headgear.
- The headgear should be easily removed. If extreme force is needed to remove it, return to the clinic to have the headgear adjusted.
- Avoid play while wearing the headgear.
- Report any headgear related injuries immediately, particularly if the injury occurs in the eye region.

Care of appliances

Care of (fixed and removable) orthodontic appliances is very important for the following reasons:
- Produce the best possible result.
- Avoid injury.
- Lower the risk of damage to the appliance.
- Avoid extending treatment.

▶ Patients must be advised to attend regular appointments and report any problems, before their routine appointment, if appropriate.

Fixed appliances

Fixed orthodontic appliances make routine oral hygiene procedures difficult and the patient is therefore more vulnerable to plaque stagnation areas. This in turn can cause:
- Enamel damage—e.g. decalcification and/or caries.
- Periodontal damage—e.g. gingivitis.

This is preventable if the patient takes good care of their appliance.

Irritation of soft tissues

Following the initial placement of the appliance, irritation and ulceration of soft tissues might occur from the sharp distal ends of archwires and steel ligatures. To limit discomfort, patients should be supplied with soft relief wax and advised to contact their orthodontist for advice.

Pain and discomfort

Patients should be advised that they are likely to experience some pain and discomfort in their teeth following placement of the appliance and may feel loose when they start moving. This could last for 1–3 days and might occasionally require painkillers. A soft diet during this period should be helpful.

Breakage of appliances

To limit the risk of breakages, patients should be advised to modify their diet and to avoid the following:
- Chewing gum, toffees, or hard foods (e.g. nuts and crusty bread).
- Biting into hard foods—e.g. apples and carrots.

Patients should be advised to contact their orthodontist in the case of a breakage and not to wait until their next routine appointment.

Sport injuries

Patients should be advised to use a protective mouthguard during contact sports; this is available from their orthodontist.

Maintenance of appliances

Patients should be advised to clean both the teeth and appliance after each meal using a normal tooth brush and a mirror to make sure all particles have been removed. Advice and instruction on how to use interdental brushes, disclosing tablets, and mouthwash to maintain good oral hygiene should also be give to the patient.

Removable appliances

Appliance wear

Patients are instructed to wear their appliance full time, except for cleaning and playing contact sports. This prevents loss and damage of the appliance.

Storage of appliances

Patients should be instructed to store appliances safely in robust boxes when they are not being worn.

Pain and discomfort

Patients should be advised that they are likely to experience some pain and discomfort in their teeth following placement of the appliance. This could last for 1–3 days and does not usually require painkillers.

Maintenance of appliances

Patients are instructed to remove their appliance for cleaning. It is important that the teeth, gums, and appliance are cleaned thoroughly to prevent damage. Appliances should be cleaned after meals by use of a toothbrush and toothpaste, taking care not to damage the brace.

Oral hygiene advice

The importance of optimal oral hygiene and general dental condition before the commencement of orthodontic treatment cannot be overemphasized. Patients who cannot keep their mouths clean before treatment are certainly not going to do so during treatment with an appliance, which collects food debris and acts as stagnation areas attracting plaque.

In particular, fixed orthodontic appliances make routine oral hygiene procedures difficult and the patient is therefore vulnerable to plaque-related disease:
• Enamel damage—e.g. decalcification and/or caries.
• Periodontal damage—e.g. gingivitis.

Plaque-related disease is preventable by maintaining good oral hygiene. If an orthodontist feels that a patient is not following a meticulous oral hygiene routine they may chose to debond a fixed appliance because of the risk poor oral hygiene can have on otherwise healthy teeth.

Oral hygiene instructions should be given with dietary advice, to prevent tooth damage (decalcification, caries, or acid erosion). In particular, intake of the following should be eliminated or restricted to meal times:
• Carbonated drinks—if carbonated drinks are consumed, the use of a straw should be encouraged, to limit contact with the teeth.
• Concentrated fruit juices.
• Retentive sweets—e.g. toffee.
• Chocolate.

Full oral hygiene advice can be found in Chapter 12.

Drugs and materials used in dentistry

Disinfectants

Definition

A disinfectant is defined as a substance that kills pathogens, working in a similar way to sterilizing agents, which destroy or remove all forms of viruses, bacteria, and fungi.

Background

Disinfectants are used externally to kill or prevent the growth of microbes and also used for disinfection of non-living surfaces, such as worktops, and items, such as impressions.

They are poisonous so should not be taken internally.

Uses

Disinfectants are mainly used in the following circumstances in the dental surgery:
- If autoclaving cannot be used, such as on work surfaces, or for items made of plastic etc. that cannot withstand the heat of an autoclave.
- In the form of a liquid soap.
- To disinfect surfaces of the skin and mouth before an injection is given.
- Disinfecting root canals during endodontic treatment.

To maintain their effectiveness, disinfectants should be made up and used in accordance with the manufacturer's instructions. Disinfection is done by using chlorhexidine, gluteraldehyde, or sodium hypochlorite solutions. There are many proprietary brands containing these substances.

Sodium hypochlorite
- Effective against the hepatitis B virus (HBV) and the human immunodeficiency virus (HIV).
- Used to disinfect work surfaces.
- Used in laboratory work, including impressions.
- Used for blood stains.

❶ Chlorhexidine can occasionally cause contact dermatitis, but it is rarely an allergen.

❶ Gluteraldehyde can irritate the eyes, skin, and respiratory tract. It might also cause other adverse reactions, such as contact dermatitis, and can also stain.

❶ Sodium hypochlorite can irritate the skin and cause serious damage to the eyes. It corrodes metals, bleaches fabrics, and discolours plastics. Only use these chemicals in well-ventilated areas and avoid contact with the skin through the use of adequate PPE.

Antiseptic agents

Definition
Similar to disinfectants, these agents are used to eliminate infection of living surfaces, such as the skin or mucosa.

Background
Some antiseptic agents can kill micro-organisms (bactericidal), whereas others only inhibit their growth (bacteriostatic).

Uses
Different types of antiseptics are used in the dental surgery:
- Alcohols used to clean skin before an injection.
- Chlorhexidine gluconate used on both the skin and the oral mucosa.
- Hydrogen peroxide used for cleaning wounds and ulcers.
- Iodine-based products for cleaning wounds.
- Benzalkonium-containing products used for cleaning the skin before surgery.

Chlorhexidine (Hibitane®)
This agent is used at different strengths for different purposes (Table 17.1).

Tincture of iodine
A solution of iodine can be used to disinfect the skin or mouth surface before an injection and marks the area with a brownish colouring. It is used for intraosseous and intraligamentary injections and disinfecting the gingival crevice before an extraction.

Hydrogen peroxide
This agent is used at different strengths for different purposes (Table 17.2). It is the best choice for acute ulcerative gingivitis (AUG).

Table 17.1 Chlorhexidine strengths and uses

Solution	Uses
0.2%	Antiseptic mouthwash
0.5%	Disinfecting skin or mouth surfaces before an injection
1% gel	Used if oral ulceration inhibits brushing of teeth, keeps the oral cavity clean, and prevents formation of plaque

Table 17.2 Hydrogen peroxide strengths and uses

Solution	Uses
0.5%	Cleansing and deodorant mouthwash
3%	Irrigating dry sockets

Antibacterial agents

Definition

Antibacterial agents are taken internally to kill bacteria.

Uses

The most common dental uses for an antibacterial drug are to treat an acute alveolar abscess or rise in temperature. In dentistry, they are also of great importance in the treatment of patients who are at risk of endocarditis. See Table 17.3.

Prescription of antibacterial agents

This category includes antibiotics and metronidazole.

Penicillin and its derivatives are common drugs, which people are sometimes allergic to. If prescribed to an allergic patient, these agents could cause a severe allergic reaction. It is important that a patient's medical history is thoroughly checked before treatment is prescribed, to check for any allergies, current medications, and risk of endocarditis.

Table 17.3 Antibacterial agents

Drug	Uses
Penicillin	Can be administered by injection or mouth
	Prevention of the spread of infection in pericoronitis, cellulitis, and jaw fractures
	Prevention of wound infections following minor oral surgery
	Has a severe adverse reaction if given with methotrexate, which is often used in cancer treatment and cases of severe psoriasis
Amoxicillin	Derivative of penicillin
	Given by mouth
	Taken for infections not responding to penicillin
	Antibiotic cover
Erythromycin	Given by mouth
	Prescribed to patients allergic to both penicillin and amoxicillin or for infections resistant to both these agents
Clindamycin	Given by mouth
	Antibiotic cover if the patient is allergic to penicillin or its derivatives
Tetracycline	Given by mouth or external application (mouthwash)
	Relieves discomfort from recurrent ulcers that have not responded to other drugs
	Local application to gingival pockets in periodontal disease
	Might cause permanent discoloration if taken internally while teeth are still being formed
	If taken in pregnancy it could affect the deciduous dentition in an unborn child
	Might affect the permanent teeth of a child <12 years old
	Permanent damage can also occur in those who receiving long-term tetracycline treatment
Metronidazole (Flagyl®)	Given by mouth
	Used for treatment of acute ulcerative gingivitis and pericoronitis and in those allergic to penicillin or its derivatives
	Alcohol should be avoided while taking metronidazole
	Should not be prescribed during pregnancy, breastfeeding, or for patients taking cyclosporin (a cancer drug) or some antiepileptic drugs.

Antibiotic cover and prophylaxis

Definition

In dentistry, 'antibiotic cover' is the use of antibiotic agents to prevent endocarditis in at-risk patients.

Bacteraemia and infective endocarditis

Bacteraemia is a transient presence of bacteria or other micro-organisms in the blood. It can lead to infective endocarditis, a rare but dangerous condition affecting the internal surface lining of the heart called the 'endocardium'.

The infection affects mostly the heart valves, especially damaged ones. Damaged heart valves can lead to turbulent blood flow, which, in turn, can lead to the formation of deposits of platelets and fibrin called 'vegetations' on the damaged valves. These vegetations can readily become infected following bacteraemia.

The most significant bacteria are *Streptococcus mutans* and *Streptococcus sanguis*, which are found in dental plaque.

Preventing bacteraemia and infective endocarditis

- A careful history must be taken.
- The following preventative measures should be taken:
  - Identification of patients at risk.
  - Improving patients' oral hygiene before dental treatment.

At-risk patients

- Those who have had endocarditis in the past.
- Those who have had heart surgery.
- Those with damaged or artificial heart valves.
- Those who are immunocompromised.

Prophylaxis

You may be aware that NICE published new national guidelines on antibiotic prophylaxis for the prevention of endocarditis in 2009.[1]

Essentially: antibiotic prophylaxis against infective endocarditis should no longer be offered for *any* patients undergoing any dental procedures, including those patients considered at risk for infective endocarditis.

Furthermore, chlorhexidine mouthwash should *not* be used as prophylaxis against infective endocarditis in people at risk undergoing dental procedures.

It is important that patients are aware of the importance of maintaining good oral health, and those patients at risk of infective endocarditis should be advised that antibiotic prophylaxis is no longer routinely recommended.

---

[1] NICE (2008). *Antibiotic prophylaxis against infective endocarditis*. London: NICE. Available at: ℘ http://guidance.nice.org.uk/CG64.

Analgesic agents

Definition
Analgesics relieve pain.

Uses
These agents have a more limited effect compared with anaesthetics that remove pain and other sensations altogether. Analgesics can be local or systemic (see Chapter 18).

Local analgesics
These are the drugs most commonly used in dental practice. A local analgesic solution is injected into oral tissues before dental treatment. The solution numbs the nerves so that pain is no longer felt. However, the patient can feel touch. The extent of analgesia depends on the site of the injection and whether a major nerve or branch of a nerve is affected.

The analgesic agent (usually lignocaine or similar substance), a vasoconstrictor (in the form of adrenaline [epinephrine] or felypressin) to reduce blood flow, and a preservative (sodium bisulphite) to prolong the life of the agent are contained in normal or physiological saline. The solution is supplied in 2.2mL cartridges for use with a syringe.

There are many brands available so it is important to be familiar with them and their respective concentrations.

Surface analgesics
These drugs are similar to local analgesics, except they are in the form of a paste that can be applied to the skin or mucosa to numb the surface. These agents are most commonly applied at the site of an injection to minimize the pain a patient might suffer when an injection needle enters the mucosa.

Systemic analgesics
Most patients suffer dental pain because of inflammation of the pulp ('pulpitis') or periodontium ('periodontitis') or disorders of the temporomandibular joint. It is very common to give non-steroidal anti-inflammatory drugs because of their associated analgesic properties. However, prescription of systemic analgesics (e.g. aspirin, paracetamol, ibuprofen, codeine, and pethidine) must be combined with treatment of the causes of dental pain.

Role of the dental nurse

▶ All analgesics can be dangerous if abused

▶ It is important to be familiar with the drugs by reading the information supplied with each:
• Indications.
• Contraindications.
• Adverse reactions.
• Maximum safe doses of each drug.

Although local analgesics control pain locally, they can have systemic effects. They can affect the heart and depress the cardiovascular system. At the same time, the central nervous system can be stimulated. At high doses, these agents can depress the respiratory system. It is important not to exceed the maximum safe dose:

- 2% lignocaine with adrenaline—8 cartridges.
- 3% prilocaine with felypressin—6 cartridges.

Tip

Keep count of the number of cartridges used. To this end, the empty cartridges should not be discarded until the patient has left the surgery.

Other drugs used in the dental surgery

Antifungal agents

Uses

Antifungal drugs are used in dentistry to treat *Candida albicans* fungal infections, such as the following:
- Denture stomatitis—denture sore mouth.
- Thrush.
- Angular cheilitis—soreness at the angle of the mouth.

Prescription of antifungal agents

Antifungal drugs can be prescribed in a gel form or as pastilles or lozenges:
- Nystatin —commonly pastilles.
- Miconazole—Daktarin® gel.

Sodium hypochlorite is also used to eliminate *C. albicans* from dentures by immersing them in a solution overnight.

> ❶ Miconazole should not be prescribed to the following people:
> - Patients taking anticoagulants.
> - Expectant mothers.
> - Breastfeeding mothers.

Antiviral agents

Herpes is an example of a virus affecting the mouth and the face.

HIV is in a class of its own (known as 'retroviruses') for which there is no known treatment—drugs only control the symptoms. Although there have been several reported cases of dental staff contracting HIV from patients, there has been only 1 case of a patient contracting HIV from a dentist. HIV is usually acquired by exchange of body fluids. However, every precaution must be taken to minimize the risk of transmission.

Prescription of antiviral agents

In general, viral infections must be treated systemically, although some topical treatment is also given. Acyclovir is widely used, but there are more recently introduced agents available.

Anti-inflammatory agents

Uses

These are drugs that suppress inflammation and relieve symptoms, such as pain, fever, swelling, and redness.

Prescription of anti-inflammatory agents

Steroids are used in a variety of forms:
- Topical—surface application.
- Oral—systemic use.
- Parenteral—injection.

Ledermix® (a topical paste) is used to suppress pulpal pain.

Hydrocortisone and its derivatives are marketed as lozenges, creams, paste, tablets, ointments, and sprays.

Adverse effects

Long-term systemic use can lead to deficient functioning of adrenal glands.

Haemostatic agents

Systemic corticosteroids are used for prophylaxis in patients with deficient functioning of adrenal glands. Hydrocortisone is also a drug used for emergency resuscitation. It is a legal requirement for dental workers to be competent in emergency resuscitation.

Uses

Bleeding can occur after injury to the skin or mucosa. In healthy individuals, bleeding is controlled by coagulation or clotting of the blood. However, in some individuals there might be a defect in the clotting mechanism, leading to prolonged bleeding:

- Haemophiliacs.
- Patients who have been put on anticoagulant therapy, such as warfarin, to prevent excessive clotting of the blood.

These patients can also suffer prolonged bleeding after injury or surgery. One of the components of a blood clot is fibrin, which can be dissolved or lysed, leading to bleeding.

Prescription of haemostatic agents

Haemostatic agents, such as tranexamic acid, can be used to control bleeding after a tooth extraction in susceptible patients.

Role of the dental nurse

❶ A patient's medical history must be carefully checked before dental treatment to ensure that the patient is not suffering from any bleeding disorder or on warfarin therapy. Nurses have an important role in this regard.

The surgery should also stock haemostatic agents.

Amalgam

Ingredients

Amalgam alloy consists of silver, tin, copper, and zinc. When mixed with mercury, this alloy sets as 'amalgam', a material used to restore posterior teeth.

Some newer amalgam alloys do not contain zinc because it can result in the expansion of amalgam if contaminated with saliva. However, they have higher levels of copper to ↑ strength and durability.

Properties

Amalgam is strong, durable, radio-opaque, and forgiving in terms of moisture control. However, it is metallic, conductive to heat and cold, and not adhesive.

The initial set takes 7–10 minutes, with the final set taking 24 hours.

Using amalgam

Amalgam is a restorative filling material commonly used in dentistry.

Cavities should be undercut for retention. Dentine pins can be used to assist retention of large cavities for which large parts of the crown of the tooth are missing (see 📖 Amalgam restorations, p.266).

Procedure

The alloy and mercury are mixed together using an amalgamator, according to the recommended manufacturer's instructions. Most modern day practices used repacked disposable capsules that contain the correct ratio of alloy and mercury. These capsules help prevent mercury spillage. Correct preparation is essential to prevent weakness, expansion, or contraction so the manufacturer's instructions must be followed at all times.

Advantages

Amalgam is very simple to use and the cost of the material is relatively cheap. It is strong and durable and can be placed in posterior teeth because it can withstand the forces of mastication.

Disadvantages

Because of its silvery colour, amalgam is not aesthetically pleasing so is not used in anterior teeth. Amalgam is also a conductor of temperature so cavities (unless very shallow) should be lined with a suitable material to help protect the pulp against thermal shock.

Precautions

Precautions must be taken when handling amalgam because mercury is a hazardous chemical and should be handled with care:

- Full PPE must be worn at all times to prevent mercury being absorbed by the body.
- Waste amalgam must be stored in special containers obtained from specialist companies, which will also collect the containers regularly for safe disposal.
- The current practice of supplying alloy and mercury in sealed capsules makes handling safer.
- The removal of old fillings presents the greatest risk of producing mercury vapour—high-volume suction with an amalgam filter must be used.

Tips

- If special containers are unavailable, the waste amalgam should be stored under water until safe disposal, to minimize the risk of mercury vapour drifting into the workplace.
- Do not throw waste amalgam into sinks.

Mercury poisoning

❶ Mercury is a poisonous substance that can cause serious damage to the human body.

Exposure

Mercury can be absorbed through direct contact with the skin or its vapour can be inhaled. It can also be absorbed when amalgam fillings are being removed—a cloud of particles is created, which can be inhaled or contaminate the eyes or skin.

Mercury vapour

Mercury vapour is extremely dangerous because it cannot be seen. Mercury and amalgam let off a vapour at normal room temperature and this vapour ↑ as the temperature rises. Both amalgam and mercury should be stored in a sealed container in a cool and well-ventilated area.

Symptoms of mercury poisoning

Early symptoms of mercury poisoning can include headache, nausea, fatigue, irritability, and diarrhoea but can often go undetected at this stage. Tremor of the hands and double vision can then follow; the final stage is kidney failure.

Precautions

Do

- Always wear PPE when handling mercury and amalgam.
- Keep the surgery well ventilated.
- Use high-speed handpieces, diamond/tungsten carbide burs, a water spray, adequate aspiration, and a rubber dam during the removal of amalgam fillings.
- Store amalgam and mercury in a sealed container in a cool, well-ventilated area. Ensure containers are well labelled and unbreakable.
- Store and handle amalgam and mercury in just one area of the surgery.
- Prepare amalgam over a drip tray to contain any spillages.
- Use repacked amalgam capsules to help prevent spillage.
- Remove all traces of amalgam from instruments before they are placed into the sterilizer.
- Take the appropriate action in the event of a mercury spillage (see 📖 Mercury spillage, p.357).

Don't

- Don't wear open-toed shoes.
- Don't wear jewellery because this can harbour particles of amalgam.
- Don't flush amalgam down sinks or spittoons.
- Avoid eating, drinking, and applying cosmetics in clinical areas because these actions could promote the absorption of mercury.
- Floor coverings should not have any cracks or gaps that could trap amalgam or mercury—carpet must not be used.

Mercury spillage

Although the current practice of supplying amalgam alloy and mercury in a sealed capsule makes this less likely, improper mixing or faulty seals on capsules can lead to mercury spillage.

Immediate action

In the event of a mercury spillage, the following actions should be taken:
- Report the spillage to the dentist or senior nurse immediately.
- Isolate the area.
- Provide ventilation.
- Put on PPE.

Clearing up

Small spills
- See Table 17.4. Mercury spillage kits are also available for clearing.

Table 17.4 Cleaning methods for mercury spillages

Mercury appearance	Cleaning method
Waste amalgam	Collect using a damp paper towel
Globules	Mercury can be drawn up into an intravenous syringe or bulb aspirator and transferred to a mercury container
Smaller globules	Can be absorbed using a lead foil from an x-ray film packet
Very small or numerous globules	A mercury-absorbent paste made of calcium oxide, flowers of sulphur, and water can be smeared over the area. This is left to dry, then removed with a wet paper towel

Large spills
- The health and safety executive (HSE) must be informed.
- Records of the incident and its outcome should be recorded in the practice incident/accident book.
- Commercial spillage kits, which contain the items needed, are available to buy and many modern practices have these or put their own together.
- If there is reason to believe there is mercury contamination in the surgery, a test can be carried out to see how much mercury vapour is in the air. Staff can also be tested at the hospital to see whether they have absorbed dangerous amounts of mercury.

▶ Precautions

- On no account should spilled mercury be 'swept under the carpet' or put into waste bins or sinks.
- Never use a vacuum cleaner or aspirator to collect the spillage because they can vapourize the mercury and discharge it into the air.

Glass ionomer cement

Ingredients

Glass ionomer is supplied as a powder of aluminosilicate glass. When mixed with a polyacid, this becomes the set material. Initially, the glass ionomer powder and polyacid liquid were supplied in separate bottles. However, current practice is to freeze dry the polyacid, add it to the aluminosilicate glass powder, and supply both in the same bottle. The bottle of liquid supplied contains only deionized water. The powder must be mixed with the water to activate freeze-dried polyacid particles.

Properties

The adhesive properties and 'tooth' colour of glass ionomer cement make it a suitable material for cervical abrasion cavities. The presence of fluoride confers cariostatic properties.

With a mixing time of 20 seconds, the glass ionomer restorative material sets in about 20 minutes. However, the final set takes 24 hours, during which time the material must be protected from contamination by moisture and dehydration by covering it with a layer of composite resin. Varnish is also used but is less effective.

Using glass ionomer cement

(Also see 📖 Glass ionomer restorations, p.270.)

Since its introduction in the 1970s, glass ionomer cement has undergone considerable change. It is now available as a restorative material, in addition to a luting cement. Chemically, there are the following variants:
- Resin-modified varieties.
- Glass ionomer combinations—composite compomers.

Glass ionomer luting cement is used for cementing crowns, inlays, onlays, bridges, and orthodontic bands. It has finer particles to ensure the smooth flow of material necessary during cementation. Its mixing time is about 15 seconds and the initial set takes twice as long as the restorative type glass ionomer cement.

Resin-modified variants can be cured by exposure light in the same way as composites.

Precautions
- Do not use tap water to mix glass ionomer powder if the bottle of deionized water is empty.
- Do not mix different varieties of glass ionomer cement together.

Composites

Ingredients

These are resin polymers that have revolutionized cosmetic dentistry.

Properties

Composites come in a variety of presentations, as follows:
- Chemically cured composite—sets when base and catalyst pastes are mixed.
- Light-cured composite—a photo-sensitive paste that sets when exposed to light of a particular wavelength. In dental practices, a blue light is commonly used.
- Dual-cure composite—the setting reaction is activated by a light but continues with a chemical reaction. This type of composite is used for cementing veneers, to ensure complete setting of the material.

Uses

(Also see 📖 Composite restorations, p.268.)

They are the same colour as teeth and, with light-curing techniques, can be used for the following purposes:
- To restore both anterior and posterior teeth.
- Recontouring teeth.
- As facings or veneers on discoloured teeth.
- To build up a grossly destroyed tooth ('core build up') before placing a crown.

Cements

There are a variety of cements available as outlined her.

Temporary cements

Zinc oxide eugenol (ZOE) cement

This is used as a temporary restorative material and also a lining material under amalgam restorations. It comes as a zinc oxide (ZnO) powder and eugenol liquid. The components are mixed for 1 minute and the material sets within 4–5 minutes. Setting can be accelerated by dabbing the restoration with moist cotton wool.

Reinforced ZOE cement

This is used as a long-term temporary restorative material and a lining under restorations. The powder and liquid are mixed for 1 minute and the material sets within 5 minutes.

Do not use ZOE cement under composite restorations because it affects the composite.

Temporary cement

This material is used to cement a crown temporarily. It is a ZOE-based cement, which comes as a 2-paste system of a base and catalyst. The components are mixed for 30 seconds and the material sets within 3 minutes. It is strong but easy to remove.

Permanent cements

Zinc phosphate cement

This material is used for permanent cementation of crowns, inlays, onlays, and bridges. It can also be used as a temporary restorative material because it is stronger than ZOE cement.

It comes as a ZnO powder and phosphoric acid liquid. The components are mixed for 90 seconds and the material sets in 5–8 minutes. Because of the presence of phosphoric acid, this cement cannot be used in deep cavities because it can irritate the pulp.

Zinc polycarboxylate cement

This material is used for permanent cementation of inlays, onlays, crowns, and bridges. It is also used to cement orthodontic bands and as a temporary restorative material. It is strong and adhesive.

It comes as a powder and liquid, which take 13 seconds to mix and 6 minutes to set.

Because of its adhesive properties, the material tends to stick to instruments.

Calcium hydroxide cement

This is variously termed a 'cement', 'liner', or 'base'. It is biocompatible, promotes healing, and, because it is alkaline, kills bacteria. This type of cement is used in deep cavities as a liner and also for pulp capping.

It comes as a 2-paste system of a base and catalyst. The components are mixed for 10 seconds and the material sets in 1–2 minutes.

The cement is not strong and therefore not used as a temporary restorative material. Unlike ZOE cement, it can be used under composite restorations.

Etchants

These are acids used to etch enamel before bonding composite. They dissolve enamel to leave a porous surface suitable for bonding.

Ingredients

The acid most commonly used is phosphoric acid. Some etchants have other acids added to phosphoric acid at a strength of 30–50%, with the most common concentration being 37%.

Phosphoric acid etchants were initially supplied as a clear liquid. However, this made exact placement of the etchant on a specific area difficult to see. Nowadays, the acid is incorporated into a coloured gel and presented as a paste.

Using etchants

The etchant is applied to the enamel surface for 20–30 seconds and then the surface is thoroughly washed and dried before the composite is applied. Proper etching causes enamel to lose its shine, giving rise to a dull, frosted appearance. The gel is more difficult to wash than the liquid but the colour helps to recognize unwashed, residual gel.

Precautions

Avoid contact with soft tissues.

Temporary materials

These are materials used for making temporary inlays, onlays, crowns, and bridges. There are 2 basic types as outlined here.

Acrylic-based temporary materials

These materials are chemically similar to denture base materials. The material comes as an acrylic powder and monomer liquid. The 2 components are mixed to produce a paste, which is used to make temporary restorations.

The technique consists of taking an impression of the tooth to be prepared in silicone putty. After preparation is complete, the putty impression is filled with the mixed material and carefully reseated over the tooth. Once the material has partially set, the impression with the temporary restoration inside is carefully removed and the restoration prised free, finished, and cemented with temporary cement.

This material is an irritant to the skin and mucosa. The monomer can irritate the respiratory tract and must not be inhaled.

Resin-based temporary materials

These materials are similar to composite restorative materials. They reproduce detail better than acrylic-based materials and give a better surface finish too. However, resin-based materials are brittle and the temporary must be removed from the impression of the prepared tooth with great care.

Impression materials

These are used to make a negative likeness ('impression') of teeth. The impression is then converted to a positive likeness ('cast') by pouring either plaster of Paris or dental stone into the impression.

Alginate

This is used to make primary impressions. It consists of sodium potassium alginate, calcium sulphate, sodium phosphate, diatomaceous earth filler, modifiers, colourings, and flavourings.

The powder is mixed with water at room temperature in a rubber bowl before loading onto a tray. The setting time is 3–6 minutes.

It is a non-irritant material with a pleasant smell, taste, and low cost. However, it is dimensionally unstable: changes shape due to absorption of moisture or loses water and shrinks, so much so that the impression has to be cast within 10 minutes. Otherwise, the impression must be stored in a humid environment (e.g. by wrapping in moist gauze). It also tears easily.

Polyether

This material is used for taking final impressions for making inlays, onlays, crowns, bridges, and dentures. It comes as a 2-paste system of a base and catalyst. Correct proportioning of base and catalyst is achieved by dispensing equal lengths of the material. To help get a uniform mix, the 2 pastes are coloured differently—a proper mix is indicated by a streak-free paste. The components are mixed for 45 seconds and the material sets in 3 minutes.

More recently, polyether has been made available in cartridges that are loaded onto a special gun. As the trigger is squeezed, the material is extruded through the nozzle properly mixed.

Polyether is a stiff material and therefore difficult to remove from the mouth. It should not be used in a close-fitting special tray or in a mouth with large undercuts.

Silicone

One of the most popular materials used for taking final impressions for inlays, onlays, crowns, bridges, and dentures. It is available in 4 consistencies: light, medium, heavy, and putty. The first 3 consistencies are used for final impressions, whereas putty is used to take an impression before tooth preparation for a temporary restoration.

These materials now come in cartridges that can be loaded into a special gun similar to that used for polyether. In general, 2 consistencies are used together to get an accurate impression. The light body is syringed around the teeth and the medium or heavy body is loaded onto a tray. Once the tray is correctly seated in the mouth, the 2 consistencies set together. This technique is often referred to as the 'mixed viscosity' technique.

Some clinicians use a different technique called the 'putty wash' technique, in which an impression is taken in putty first. This impression is then used as a close-fitting tray to and a wash impression is taken with light-bodied silicone.

Be aware of the impression technique to be used by the clinician so that the appropriate equipment and materials can be made ready.

Control of pain and anxiety

Local anaesthesia

A local anaesthetic (LA) is a drug administered to a patient to numb an area being operated on so that a dental procedure can be carried out without pain. It is generally given as an injection of a solution of LA into the tissues of the mouth. Injections can be made into the buccal fold of the mucosa, the palate (infiltration), or the region of a specific nerve (nerve block). Following an infiltration injection, only a small area (1 or 2 teeth) is affected, but following a nerve block all the tissues or structures supplied by that nerve are affected. Hence, an inferior dental (ID; sometimes called 'inferior alveolar') block will anaesthetize all the lower teeth, in addition to the buccal gum, on 1 side.

Ingredients of a LA

Different types of LA are available for different purposes but all usually contain the following:

- An active anaesthetic agent.
- A vasoconstrictor.
- A preservative agent.
- Buffering agent.

These components are presented in a sodium chloride solution.

For example, 'Xylocaine® 2% with adrenaline (epinephrine) 1:80 000' contains 2% lidocaine hydrochloride monohydrate, which is the LA, and 1 in 80 000 parts of a vasoconstrictor, adrenaline. Apart from a little sodium metabisuphite preservative, the rest (and majority) of the contents is salt water. Other types of LA use different LA agents and vasoconstrictors and some are available with no vasoconstrictor ('plain').

How LAs work

There are 2 pharmacological classes of LA:

- Esters—cocaine, procaine, and benzocaine.
- Amines—lignocaine.

LAs work by blocking the conduction of nerves in the mouth, by preventing the passage of ions and preventing conduction of impulses along the nerve. Fine nerves are more easily anaesthetized than thick ones, and some structures, such as the dental pulp, can be hard to anaesthetize. As soon as the LA has been given, the circulating blood starts to carry it away to be broken down in the liver; this is why a vasoconstrictor, which reduces the blood supply in the area, can be useful. The vasoconstrictor prolongs the LA effect by shutting down small blood vessels in the injection site and also reduces bleeding. The concentration of LA in the area will normally have ↓ to half its original value within 1.5 hours.

Presentation and storage of LAs

The sterile LA solution is supplied by the manufacturer in a glass tube called a 'cartridge', individually packaged within a sealed pack. In the UK cartridges normally contain 2.2mL of solution, whereas elsewhere the amount is usually 1.8mL. At one end of the cartridge is a hub that is pierced by the needle, whereas the other end contains a rubber piston or 'bung'. The name, contents, and concentrations of the constituents, manufacturer, and expiry date are printed on the glass of the cartridge, which is usually up to 18 months when new. To avoid contamination, the cartridge should not be removed from the pack until it is to be used and should be stored out of the light. They also have to be stored away from heat. If, during summer or in warmer climates, there is a need to store the LA in the fridge, then the cartridges will need to be removed from the fridge in advance of the procedure so that they can reach room temperature before they are used.

Using LAs

The cartridge is placed into a specially designed syringe and a needle is attached. Long needles are used for ID nerve blocks and short needles are used for infiltration anaesthesia. All needles are provided in sealed sterile packs and, similar to the cartridges, must not be reused on another patient because they cannot be resterilized. Needles are provided with a plastic protective cover called a 'sheath'. Their point has a sharp bevel (angled cut) to make penetration of the mucosa gentle, and the needles are coated to help them slide through the tissues. The syringe has a plunger that, when pushed down by the dentist, forces the bung deeper into the cartridge and, provided the hub has been pierced by the needle, the LA solution out of the end of the needle. Most LA syringe systems are now 'self-aspirating'. This enables the dentist to check that the needle is not in a blood vessel before starting to inject. Releasing pressure on the plunger slightly, takes pressure off the bung, which sucks fluid back up the needle. If the needle is in a blood vessel, this will draw blood back into the cartridge and is easy to see. Injecting directly into a blood vessel is dangerous because the LA will circulate quickly around the patient's body rather than remain localized and might affect distant organs, such as the heart.

Preparing for injection of LAs with a topical analgesic

To minimize the pain of an injection when the needle pierces the mucosa, a topical anaesthetic may be used beforehand. A typical agent, Ultracare®, contains 20% benzocaine in a bubblegum-flavoured gel. To be effective, such gels must be applied on a cotton-wool roll several minutes before the injection. Keep the gel away from your own skin because sensitivity has been reported. Although topical LA sprays have been used in the past, these are generally not advised because the site of action and dose are very difficult to control.

Essential checks

The dental nurse should make the following checks on a cartridge before its use:
- Correct solution, as requested by the dentist.
- Cartridge is in date and has been stored in packaging, out of light.
- No puncture holes at the hub end.
- No visible damage to the glass.
- Solution is clear, with no discoloration, cloudy precipitation, or bubbles seen, which indicate contamination.
- Rubber bung just below end of glass—if level or sticking up above end discard.

NB Patient notes should also be checked for previous negative reactions—e.g. some patients have a bad reaction to LA containing adrenaline.

Using local anaesthesia in dentistry

Administration of LA in dentistry is, in general, a very safe procedure. In 2006, one of the two UK suppliers of LAs sold >40 million cartridges; in 1999 in the USA, >300 million dental LA injections were given, making LA administration the commonest procedure in dentistry.

The nurse's role in minimizing risks

The nurse's most important role is to ensure the safe delivery of the LA to the dentist for use (see ⌨ Local anaesthesia, p.366) and its disposal afterwards. Nowadays, most LA agents are given with the patient supine— this is particularly sensible when LAs are being given because it helps to avoid the possibility of the patient fainting during the procedure. However, it does mean that appropriate protection must be in place, especially the wearing of goggles to cover the patient's eyes. The nurse should pass the topical anaesthetic on a cotton-wool roll, ensuring that the skin or other structures are not contacted. The nurse can also help to reassure the patient during the injection and prevent the patient from making limb or body movements, which might cause the dentist to slip or have difficulty placing the needle correctly or steadily.

Hazards

The most serious and commonest potential hazard during administration of LAs in dentistry is a needlestick injury (see Chapter 5). This might affect the patient or a member of the dental team. It is clearly most serious after the LA has been given and the needle has penetrated tissue, when there is also a risk of transmission of blood-borne diseases. Apart from the medical dangers, the financial consequences of treating a needlestick injury are high. One study (2001) estimated the total cost of such an injury to a nurse at up to £3845.

The nurse can help to minimize the possibility of a needlestick injury by the following means:
- Taking great care when handling used syringes.
- In general, nurses should never handle a syringe with the needle unsheathed, because it is during disassembly and resheathing that most needlestick injuries occur (see ⌨ Hazardous Waste Regulations, p.74).
- Encouraging the use of 'safety' syringes in the practice. Systems are now available that can reduce risks greatly. The same study (2001), which was carried out in a major UK dental hospital, showed that the frequency of avoidable needlestick injuries ranges from an average of 12 per million hours worked in the 3 years before introduction to 0 per million hours worked in the 2nd year after the introduction of a safety syringe.

Emergencies

Fainting (see ⌨ Faints, p.136) is probably the commonest reaction to LAs and is not an emergency if correctly recognized. However, in all emergencies the following basic rules apply:
- Know your patient, especially their medical history—this should prewarn the dental team of any possible complications.

- You should be competent at basic life support and, in addition to the dentist, ensure that resuscitation equipment is on hand and working and emergency drugs are available and in date.
- At the first signs of any untoward reaction, dental procedures should be stopped and the patient's condition evaluated by the dentist.

Overdose

When used according to manufacturers' recommendations, overdose is extremely unlikely and probably only a risk if multiple dental extractions or very extensive periodontal or implant surgery are being undertaken or in children, who have much lower tolerance to all drugs. An overdose of lidocaine (lignocaine; Xylocaine®) causes lightheadedness, tinnitus (ringing in the ears), numbness around the mouth, a metallic taste, and double vision. Even higher doses of lidocaine might lead to tremors and grand mal seizure. Subsequent depression of the central nervous system might lead to respiratory arrest. The nurse can assist greatly in monitoring blood pressure and vital signs during such an emergency, in addition to the following:

- Secure and protect the patient's airway.
- Provide 100% oxygen through a nasal mask or assist breathing with a resuscitation bag.
- Assist with CPR, if necessary.
- If a seizure occurs, help to protect the patient from injuring themselves.

Injection into a blood vessel

If a LA (with adrenaline) is accidentally injected into a blood vessel, the patient will experience flushing of the skin, tachycardia (very fast heart rate), and nausea. Hypertension (high blood pressure) and tachycardia are caused by adrenaline.

Allergy

Patients often say they have experienced 'allergies' to LAs, but these are nearly always reactions resulting from injection into a blood vessel. Less than 1% of cases are true allergies and the number has ↓ since the use of amide-type LAs. The most common cause of a true allergic reaction to LAs is sensitivity to the preservative in the anaesthetic solution (LAs are available without preservative). Topical LAs containing benzocaine (an ester) might also be responsible for some allergies. A wide range of allergic reactions might be encountered, ranging from a mild rash to anaphylactic shock (see 🕮 Anaphylaxis, p.116).

Pre-existing medical conditions

- Knowledge of the medical history will alert the dental team.
- Patients with heart conditions should be treated with special care and solutions containing adrenaline will be best avoided.
- Patients with liver diseases might have difficulty in breaking down LAs afterwards, so particular care should be taken to avoid overdose.

Conscious sedation

Most patients are a little anxious about the prospect of dental treatment but can accept treatment with LA and careful management. Some, however, might require additional help from a range of additional techniques, including conscious sedation, particularly those who have developed a true phobia about dentistry or some part of it, e.g. a phobia of needles. Alternative methods of anxiety management are discussed later in this chapter (see 📖 Alternative methods of controlling anxiety, p.376). Conscious sedation might be helpful in treating patients who gag during dentistry but are not otherwise anxious.

Definition

Conscious sedation is a technique by which the use of a drug or drugs produces a state of depression of the central nervous system, enabling treatment to be carried out but during which verbal contact with the patient is maintained throughout. The drugs and techniques used to provide conscious sedation for dental treatment should carry a margin of safety wide enough to render loss of consciousness unlikely. The level of sedation must be such that the patient remains conscious, retains protective reflexes, and can respond to verbal commands.

Phobia

A 'phobia' is an extreme instance of anxiety that usually creates a pattern of total-avoidance behaviour, through which the patient does everything possible to avoid the threatening situation. Hence, in dentistry, phobic patients usually have a very poor attendance rate and only seek help when forced to by very severe pain or other symptoms. The patient usually realizes that their fear is irrational but feels unable to change this. When placed in the feared situation, they might suffer from a panic attack, heart palpitations, feeling sick, and/or fainting. These symptoms themselves might make the patient feel even more frightened.

Selection of patients

The 2 main areas outlined next must be considered.

Medical history

- A full medical history must be taken, with a special note of any conditions affecting the heart, lungs, or liver.
- Ask about any medications taken.
- The resting blood pressure should always be taken and recorded.

The American Society of Anesthesiologists (ASA) classifies both medical health and blood pressure, from Class I (a normal healthy patient) to Class V (a moribund patient who is not expected to survive without the operation).[1] In general UK dental practice conscious sedation would not normally be considered for patients with an ASA classification >II in either respect.

Extent of anxiety

The extent of a patient's anxiety is often measured by use of a short questionnaire, which produces an anxiety score. Corah's scale is commonly used. Scores range from 5 to 25—a patient with a score of ≥20 would be considered to be phobic, but patients with lower scores might not require conscious sedation in their management plan.

Methods of providing conscious sedation

The 2 main methods used in the UK are outlined here. Both methods are effective—intravenous sedation might be more effective but is also more invasive and its effects take longer to disperse, whereas inhalation sedation (IS) has a good safety profile, has a rapid recovery time, and does not require an escort for the patient.

IS is both safe and very useful for treating anxious patients, children, and those requiring special care for whom intravenous sedation is not recommended. However, both techniques should be approached with great care when elderly patients are considered.

Inhalation sedation

IS or 'relative analgesia' (RA) is delivered to the patient by a Quantiflex machine, which provides a mixture of oxygen and nitrous oxide. The machine cannot deliver <30% oxygen and has a mechanism that cuts off all the gases if the oxygen supply is cut. Exhaust gases are removed by a scavenging system. The patient breathes the gases though a rubber nosepiece and the sedationist adjusts the mixture, starting with 100% oxygen and raising the nitrous oxide content until the patient starts to show symptoms of becoming sedated, usually at about 25% nitrous oxide. Symptoms of sedation are as follows:
- Relaxed and drowsy.
- Slurred speech.
- Drooping eyelids.
- Might feel general 'warmth'.
- Tingling in fingers, toes, or lips.

At all times the patient is awake, responsive, and their reflexes are operating. Local anaesthesia is required, as normal, for most procedures. The patient recovers within minutes at the end of the procedure, when 100% oxygen is delivered.

Intravenous sedation

Intravenous sedation using a single sedative drug, usually midazolam, is delivered to the patient by inserting a needle into a vein in either the antecubital fossa or the back of the hand. The drug is slowly titrated while the patient is monitored, both visually and by use of a pulse oximeter, to check their blood oxygen and respiratory rate. Administration stops when signs of sedation are seen, as outlined in ⊞ Inhalation sedation, p.371. Recovery from sedation with midazolam takes many hours so the patient must be escorted home afterwards and looked after by a friend or relative. They must not drive or operate machinery for 24 hours.

Tip
- Sedated patients need careful monitoring.
- The nurse should be appropriately trained/qualified in sedation for this role.
- Dentists cannot sedate patients without a second appropriately trained person, usually the nurse, being present.

[1] ASA Physical Status Classification System. Available at: ॐ http://www.asahq.org/clinical/physicalstatus.htm.

General anaesthesia

Use of general anaesthesia (GA) is one of the ways by which dental care can be provided to patients, especially if other methods of controlling anxiety are ineffective, the procedure they are to undergo is particularly lengthy or uncomfortable, or they have special needs that mean they cannot cooperate sufficiently for care to be provided using LA and/or conscious sedation.

In the past GA was widely used in general dental practice, especially for procedures such as extractions, with the dentist themselves often acting as the anaesthetist. Latterly, a separate anaesthetist was required but demand had fallen because the need for extractions diminished and there were improvements in local anaesthesia and conscious sedation. There were also a small number of widely publicized deaths involving GA in general practice. All these factors led to the publication in 2000 by the UK Department of Health of a document entitled *A Conscious Decision*.[1] The main outcome of this was that in future no GA would be provided in general practice and any patients requiring it would require treatment in a hospital with critical care facilities.

Definition

GA is a state of total unconsciousness produced by the administration of a drug or combination of drugs (gases and/or injections) designed to produce total loss of consciousness, amnesia, and analgesia.

In this state a patient loses their normal protective reflexes so their vital responses must be carefully monitored throughout the procedure.

GA and dentistry

The use of GA in dentistry is now restricted to the hospital setting in the UK. Although GA is extremely safe in such a setting, its use should be restricted only to those groups of patient for whom dental care is impossible by any other means. All other methods of controlling pain and anxiety should be attempted for the phobic patient before GA is considered. Anxious patients who can only be treated using GA have very restricted access to dentistry. For obvious reasons, the number of times GA is administered will need to be minimized and as much dentistry as practicable performed under each GA. Because the patient is completely unconscious, there is no possibility of seeking their views on any treatment options during the procedure. For this reason, only fairly basic care can be provided and more complex forms of treatment, such as crowns and root-canal therapy, are extremely difficult to provide.

For non-phobic patients, improvements in LA and conscious sedation have meant that fewer patients now require GA for such routine procedures as 3rd molar extractions, and dentists try very hard to discourage patients from opting for GA unless absolutely necessary.

Patient selection

The following are some of the patients who might still require GA for dental procedures:

- Extremely phobic patients for whom all other methods of controlling anxiety have proved impossible.
- Children requiring multiple tooth extractions who will not tolerate LA.
- Patients requiring special care, especially those who cannot normally control involuntary movements during treatment.

[1] Department of Health (2000). *A Conscious Decision: A review of the use of general anaesthesia and conscious sedation in primary dental care.* London: Department of Health. Available at: http://www.dh.gov.uk/en/Publicationsandstatistics/Publications/PublicationsPolicyAndGuidance/DH_4074702.

Alternative methods of controlling anxiety

Because people are not born afraid of dentists, much of what makes individuals anxious about dentistry is usually as a result of life experiences related to dentistry:

- Direct personal experience of a less-than-sympathetic dentist in the past.
- Negative images of dentistry in the media.
- Talking to friends.
- Attitudes of parents or other family members.

If these influences develop into a full-blown phobia (see 📖 Phobia, p.370), individuals are likely to avoid the dentist altogether. This neglect might lead to a worsening of the individual's dental state and the associated embarrassment of showing their mouth to anyone might make going to the dentist even more difficult. If the individual does attend, they might suffer panic attacks and this experience will make them feel even worse. Neglect of teeth might also have other psychological effects, making an individual less sociable and causing them to avoid situations in which their appearance lets them down. Because fear of the unknown heightens anxiety, the longer the delay the more phobic an individual will become.

Solutions

Because fear and anxiety are generally conditioned responses, they can equally be unlearnt, although this might be a slow process. In the same way that people who have a fear of flying or spiders can be helped to tolerate their phobias, so people who are anxious about dentistry can be helped. Nearly all dentists in practice have received training in communication skills and are much better at explaining and listening to their patients than they were in the past. Some even offer anxiety counselling as part of their practice facilities.

The following general principles are recommended for minimizing anxiety:

- Adopt a whole-patient approach—treating patients as people and not just a set of teeth.
- Emphasis on a team approach—patients feel more secure if they appreciate a number of people are cooperating to help them.
- Make patients comfortable—warm, friendly surroundings and avoidance of a clinical/'hospital' feel, smell, and ambience.
- Avoid meeting patients looking like a 'lunar astronaut'—especially because heightened infection-control procedures have meant gloves, masks, and visors are normal wear.
- Allow patients to express themselves fully.
- Never use embarrassment or ridicule.
- Plan care carefully—especially if long or complex procedures are involved.
- Ensure patients are fully involved in treatment decisions about themselves and fully informed of options and alternatives.
- Build confidence by engendering trust—always be honest and never tell lies.

- Develop signalling systems—these allow the patient to stop the treatment at any time; for example, the commonest is to get them to raise their hand.
- Relaxation techniques, such as diaphragmatic breathing, muscle relaxation, or yoga, might be useful.
- Distraction techniques, such as listening to an MP3 player or wearing virtual-reality glasses, can be tried but these do have the disadvantage of hindering communication with the patient.
- Scheduling—simply ensuring anxious patients are booked in early in the morning might help, because they do not have the whole day to worry about their appointment.
- Try and determine exactly what the particular areas within dentistry a patient most dislikes are so specific help can be given—a questionnaire, such as Corah's (see 📖 Extent of anxiety, p.371), might help to identify these.

Additional help

Particularly anxious patients might need help even getting themselves to see the dentist. They can be helped by specific psychotherapy or counselling. Here, they will be encouraged to talk to the therapist about things that happened to them in the past and gradually face up to their fears. Some individuals can be helped similarly by hypnotherapy.

Experts have developed specific desensitization techniques, particularly for needle phobias. These usually involve a slow and systematic introduction of the patient to the dental injection syringe. They are told about topical anaesthetics and rub some into their gums. They are shown and allowed to hold the components of the syringe (including the needle) and, when they are ready, the syringe (with the sheath in place) is placed in their mouth. Eventually, they might be ready to accept an injection. Such a process can take some hours spread over a number of appointments but does have a good level of success.

Being a professional

Working as a dental nurse in the UK

Work settings for dental nurses

As from August 2008 to work as a dental nurse in the UK you will need to have achieved a recognized dental nurse qualification from an approved training establishment (see Chapter 1) and be registered with the GDC.

Nevertheless if you are training to become a dental nurse, you will need to be enrolled and attending a recognized course. It should be remembered that evidence of enrolment may be required.

Dental nurses work in a variety of settings. A majority of dental nurses work in general dental practices treating NHS and/or private patients. Community clinics also offer opportunities for dental nurses. These clinics may tend to provide care and support to young/anxious children and adults. They may also provide dental treatment to those patients who present with learning difficulties and/or physical disabilities, mental illness, and dental phobias. Those patients with complex medical conditions may also be treated within this setting. Community clinics may also undertake domiciliary visits and school visits which allow for a varied outlook in relation to dental nursing.

Opportunities also arise to work in dental hospitals. Hospitals tend to see a variety of different patients in various settings. Patients who require routine dental treatment are usually seen by dental undergraduates whilst more complex treatment may require the knowledge and expertise of specialists. Patients treated in a hospital may also present with complex medical histories which make treatment more difficult. Whilst the dental treatment may be the same, the preoperative care may be different from a patient who presents with no known medical problems.

Opportunities also arise in the military: the army, navy, and air force all provide dental services to their personnel both at home and wherever they are deployed in the world.

Applying for an appointment

Job vacancies or appointments are now advertised in many different places, such as the Internet, local and national newspapers, and, of course, the specialist dental press.

Some advertisements will include a job description whilst others may require a phone call or letter to gain this information.

It is wise to read this job description prior to contacting the potential employer. Many questions that you have may be answered by reading this information, such as working hours, rates of pay, and responsibilities. Only once you have read all the information should you consider making contact with the establishment offering the job. If you are phoning the employer, it is often helpful to write down any questions you have for them before you make contact—this helps you to appear confident and prepared to them. However, some jobs may require a letter to a named person. This should be completed as soon as possible to avoid missing closing dates.

Application documents

Curriculum vitae (CV)

Your CV is one of the first things that your potential employer may see. This is where you need to sell yourself and encourage the potential employer to call you for interview. An employer does not have time to read between the lines so you need to communicate effectively. Clear concise information will be required. However, ensure that it is of relevance to the employer. Information that a CV should contain will include:

Education and qualifications

These should relate to your secondary education and beyond. Ensure that you give the full qualification as this will help the employer recognize what qualifications you have. What does CSE, GCE, GCSE, AS-level all mean? This can be very confusing.

Work experience

Think about the skills that will be required for the position that you will be applying for. Do you have any previous experience either within or outside of the dental industry that makes you a good candidate for the job? E.g. in addition to your dental training you may have experience in other positions with transferable skills such as organizational skills, time management, and experience dealing with patients/customers.

Extra-curricular activities

What do you do in your spare time? Do you have any positions of authority or responsibility, such as running a sports group? Do you participate in any hobbies that require manual dexterity? This information gives the employer an idea of what you do outside of your working commitments.

General skills

Do you have any additional skills or attributes such as a driving licence, computer skills, etc.?

When writing your CV think about the presentation. Leave out irrelevant information as the employer may lose interest. Avoid lengthy, wordy CVs. You can elaborate on any information should you be called for interview. This may also form a discussion point at interview. Ensure that both spelling and grammar are correct. In the ideal world your CV should only be 1 side of an A4 sheet! This is difficult to achieve first time round so practise may be needed.

Most CVs are laid out in chronological order; however, you should remember that this does not have to be the option you choose. You should select the format which best suits the job.

Don't expect your first CV to be your best. You may need to complete a few drafts prior to sending any off to potential employers. However, remember the following:

- Do not send a CV until you are happy with it.
- Check spelling and grammar.
- Check for unnecessary material.

- Show your CV to someone who you trust. Listen to any suggestions. Constructive criticism is appreciated.
- Print on good quality paper.

Application form

Application forms now come in different formats. We find both paper and electronic versions. When completing an application form it is always best to have a spare copy.

Always make sure that you read the application form first. Sometimes dates may go from first to last or vice versa so ensure that this is understood. Be honest on the application form. If you have gaps in your employment history then this may be picked up at interview so ensure you know what you were doing at that time.

An electronic copy can be a little more difficult as it may contain drop-down boxes. Again take your time completing the form and if possible print out the form once you have completed it. You can then check your form prior to submitting.

If completing a paper application form it is best to photocopy the original first and then complete the photocopy. If you make any mistakes then you can change them on the copy without destroying the original. Once you are happy you can then transfer the information on to the original. Once complete you may wish to photocopy the original for your records prior to sending your application form.

Once you have sent your application form off you cannot do much but wait. Some establishments will write to confirm if you have been successfully short listed or not whilst some will inform you only if you have been successful.

The interview

Preparation

The interview is one of the most important parts of the process in obtaining your ideal job. So what can you do to improve your chances?

Do some research

It is not advisable to walk in to an interview without knowing a little about the practice, community, or hospital. Most practices now have websites where information can be obtained. Community centres and hospitals will have generalized websites so spend some time looking at the mission statements and local community that it serves.

Plan your route

Ensure you know exactly where you are going on the day. If possible follow the route prior to the day and work out alternatives in case of transport cancellations, increased traffic, or station closures. Plan to arrive about 15 minutes early. Should you arrive late it may be impossible to repair the damage!

Dress and appearance

Appearance counts. Dress appropriately for your interview. Jeans and tee-shirts are not appropriate and will not create the right impression. Most people will wear a suit. However, smart trousers or a skirt along with a smart top will suffice.

Be prepared

Be prepared for the unexpected. You never know what an interview panel will ask, however you should be prepared for any question. This will help you demonstrate your ability to think and answer on the spot. A popular question would be 'What are your strengths?'. Most people can answer this without thinking, nevertheless, if asked 'What are your weaknesses?' this can be a much more difficult question to answer!

Ensure you know the plan for the interview. Will you be required to carry out any practical tests? Will you be required to complete a written assessment? Any additional information with regards to the interview should be sent to you with the invitation to interview.

Questions

It is always advisable to have a few questions prepared for the interview panel. Prepare 1 or 2 questions about the specific job, organization, or possible career progression. These questions may arise from reading the job description.

So what happens at the interview?

You must prove to the interview panel in a face-to-face meeting that you have the credentials, personality, and experience to carry out the job.

First impressions

As soon as you walk into the room, the interview panel is making assumptions about you. This can be a difficult time as you see your panel for the first time. It is important to remember that at an interview at a dental practice only the principal dentist and possibly the practice manager and/ or senior dental nurse may be present. A hospital or community may have a larger panel, sometimes up to 4 people.

Try to display a calm, friendly, but professional manner. The shaking of individuals hands is very much a personal choice. Be guided by the lead interviewer to a chair and then take a seat.

Eye contact

Try to maintain eye contact with the interviewer who is asking the questions. It is easy for eyes to start wandering when a difficult or unexpected question is asked. If being interviewed by more than 1 interviewer, then direct your answers to the interviewer asking the question. Once you have given your answer you can then look to the other interviewers.

Questions

Keep your answers to questions short and to the point but make sure you answer the question. Should the interviewers want additional information, they will ask.

Body language

Your body language can give a lot away without you really knowing. Try to sit in a comfortable position and avoid crossing your arms or legs during the interview. This can create a potential barrier. Hands should be neatly placed in your lap.

Post-registration education

Lifelong learning

The philosophy behind lifelong learning is that it we continue to learn throughout our professional lives. This learning may take the form of distance learning courses, e-learning courses, further education, and correspondence courses.

Continuing professional development

As from 1 August 2008, DCPs will be required to complete and record 150 hours of CPD every 5 years. 1/3 of this (50 hours) must be verifiable.

Verifiable CPD

The activity/course must have:
- Educational aims and objectives.
- A clearly defined outcome.
- An opportunity to give feedback on the activity.

You should also keep proof and/or certificate of attendance.

Non-verifiable CPD

This may include journal reading. Some journals have sections that you can complete and return once you have completed a short quiz.

Post-qualification courses

Post-qualification certificate courses are offered covering a variety of topics. Additional 1-day courses are also run which may be of great benefit to dental nurses. These courses can be found in dental journals and sometimes on deanery websites.

Certificate in oral health education

This qualification will allow the dental nurse to confidently give patients from a wide spectrum of the community, advice on oral health. This would be an ideal qualification for those interested in oral health promotion.

Certificate in dental sedation

This qualification should be considered for those interested in conscious sedation. The course covers all aspects of sedation techniques and patient care. This will ensure that nurses assisting clinicians with sedation techniques are properly trained.

Certificate in special care dental nursing

This qualification is suitable for those dental nurses who work and assist with patients whose health and care needs may require additional oral healthcare provision, e.g. those with medically compromising conditions such as bleeding disorders, or those with physical disabilities who are confined to a wheel chair.

Certificate in orthodontic nursing

This is a worthwhile course to undertake especially if you would like to specialize in an orthodontic practice. This will also help should you wish to consider the Orthodontic Therapy course.

Dental radiography
The taking of radiographs in any dental surgery is a routine procedure. Dental nurses now have the ability to legally take radiographs after undertaking an approved course of training and passing the approved examination.

Certificate in education
Any dental nurse who is considering teaching should consider the certificate in education. The certificate in education provides a good foundation for those who have an interest in education and the delivery of dental nurse training.

The Diploma in Teaching in the Lifelong Learning Sector (DTLLS) has since replaced the full Cert Ed; however, as a start, dental nurses interested in teaching can work towards Preparing to teach in the Lifelong Learning Sector (PTLLS).

Depending on the experience levels the Certificate in Teaching in the Lifelong Learning Sector (CTLLS) may be an alternative option.

Each course should be looked into and then the most appropriate one selected to meet the need of both the dental nurse and teaching establishment.

Foundation degree in dental nursing
This is a new qualification that dental nurses can undertake once they have qualified. Whilst the qualification contains some of the post-qualification courses, it is at a higher academic level.

The opportunities once qualified as a dental nurse are changing all the time; however, these are just some of the career paths available:
- Oral health educator/promoter.
- Practice manager.
- Lead/Senior dental nurse.
- Infection control nurse.
- Telephone dental nurse advisor (NHS Direct).
- Dental nurse trainer/assessor (related to the NVQ).
- Dental hygienist/therapist (further training).
- Orthodontic nursing.
- Orthodontic therapist.

Dental instrument identification

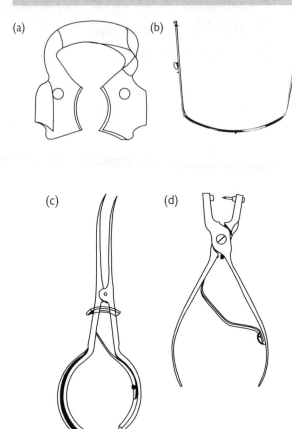

Fig. A.1 Rubber dam equipment comprising: (a) rubber dam clamp; (b) metal rubber dam frame; (c) rubber dam clamp forceps; (d) rubber dam hole punch.

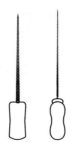

Fig. A.2 Root canal files.

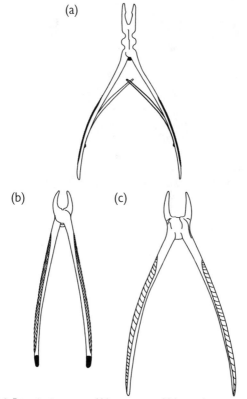

Fig. A.3 Extraction instruments: (a) bone rongeurs; (b) forceps (upper centrals, canines, and roots); (c) forceps (upper premolars and roots).

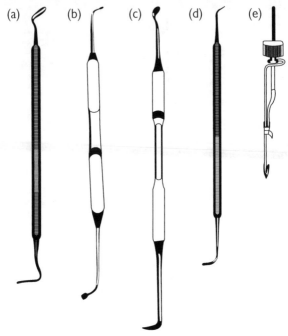

Fig. A.4 Instruments for conveying, placing, and shaping composite materials:
(a) flat plastic instrument; (b) plugger; (c) Mitchells (osteo) trimmer; (d) burnisher;
(e) Siqveland matrix retainer.

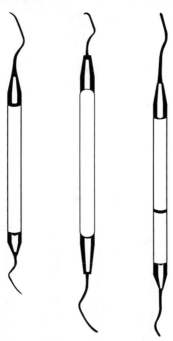

Fig. A.5 Hand-held periodontal scalers, used to remove supra- and sub-gingival calculus deposits.

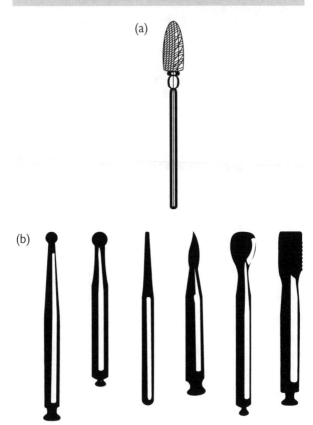

Fig. A.6 Burs: (a) acrylic trimming bur for a straight handpiece; (b) from left to right: small round bur; large round bur; tapered fissure bur; flame; pear; inverted cone.

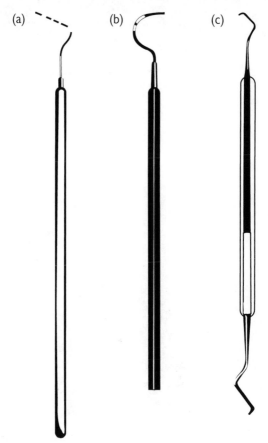

Fig. A.7 Dental probes (round-ended) for periodontal examination and assessing roughness of enamel/occlusal surfaces and (sharp) for checking restoration margins and carious dentine to be excavated: (a) Williams' probe (periodontal pocket measuring probe); (b) sickle probe; (c) Briault probe.

Index

Printed and bound by CPI Group (UK) Ltd, Croydon, CR0 4YY